PREVENTING AUTOMOBILE INJURY

PREVENTING AUTOMOBILE INJURY

New Findings from Evaluation Research

Edited by
JOHN D. GRAHAM
Harvard School of Public Health

Auburn House Publishing Company
Dover, Massachusetts

363.125
P944

Library of Congress Cataloging in Publication Data

Preventing automobile injury.

    Includes proceedings of a conference convened in Boston by the
New England Injury Prevention Research Center, Dec. 10–11, 1987.
    Includes index.
    1. Traffic safety—Congresses. I. Graham, John D.
(John David), 1956–   . II. New England Injury
Prevention Research Center.
HE5614.P747   1988   363.1′257   88-14636
ISBN 0-86569-185-1

Printed in the United States of America

FOREWORD

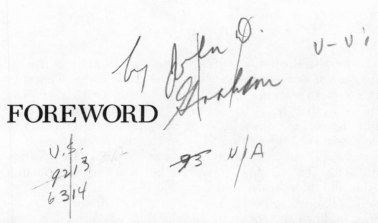

Preventing Automobile Injury is the first major product of the New England Injury Prevention Research Center (NEIPRC). The significance of this volume lies not only in its excellent content but also in the fact that it results from an emerging national recognition of the magnitude of the injury problem and the need to stimulate new thinking and research on both the prevention and treatment of injuries.

Current interest in injury prevention was stimulated by publication of *Injury in America: A Continuing Public Health Problem,* by the Committee on Trauma Research of the Institute of Medicine. A major argument put forward by the Committee was that funding for research on injury prevention is not consonant with the magnitude of the problem. While injury accounts for more years of productive life lost than either cancer or heart disease in this country, it receives less than 2 percent of federal biomedical research funds. As a result, Congress and the Centers for Disease Control (CDC) have created five new injury prevention research centers throughout the country to stimulate research, teach professionals about the public health aspects of injury, pinpoint prevention opportunities, and place this problem on the national agenda.

The New England Injury Prevention Research Center is one of the five national centers. The NEIPRC is a collaborative effort of the Harvard School of Public Health, Boston University Schools of Medicine and Public Health, Tufts University Medical School and College of Engineering, The Educational Development Center, and the Massachusetts Department of Public Health. A multidisciplinary faculty is involved in three major areas of research: unintentional injuries to children, violence and intentional injury, and motor-vehicle-related injury. Several NEIPRC faculty participated in the December 1987 research conference and contributed to this volume. We believe that *Preventing Automobile Injury* fulfills the best intent of the Committee, the Congress, CDC, and the National Highway Traffic Safety Administration (NHTSA).

v

The chapters in this book represent the current state of the art in evaluation research on motor-vehicle-related injury and point to numerous effective countermeasures. A major message of the conference was that the safety research community must critically reexamine the role of human behavior in injury prevention. Sound scientific evidence is presented to show that behavior change, as well as technological innovation, is a feasible and cost-effective approach. The final chapter reframes the issue into a research agenda that should be addressed in the future.

The NEIPRC welcomes the opportunity to disseminate the conference findings and congratulates the authors on the quality of their contributions. Dr. John Graham did a marvelous job as organizer and editor in bringing together the leaders of the field to highlight successes of the past and challenges for the future.

BERNARD GUYER, MD MPH

Associate Professor of Maternal and Child Health,
and Director, New England Injury Prevention Research Center,
Harvard School of Public Health, Boston

ACKNOWLEDGMENTS

This book is the product of an invitational research conference, "Preventing Motor Vehicle Injuries," convened in Boston by the New England Injury Prevention Research Center (NEIPRC) on December 10 and 11 of 1987. The conference was organized by a steering committee comprised of Leonard Evans (General Motors Corporation), Barry Felrice (National Highway Traffic Safety Administration), John D. Graham (Harvard School of Public Health), Ralph Hingson (Boston University School of Public Health), Cheryl Vince (Educational Development Center), and Allan Williams (Insurance Institute for Highway Safety). The purpose of the conference was to assess recent "evaluation research" about traffic safety policy.

In order to foster lively and relevant discussion, conference participants were drawn from multiple disciplines and included advocates and policymakers as well as researchers. The book itself includes an introduction to the field, the major papers presented at the conference, the prepared comments of conference discussants, and an analysis of research and policy directions based on deliberations at the conference.

The findings in Chapter 7 of this book are based on the oral remarks of participants at the conference. In addition to the contributors to this book, conference participants included Joan Claybrook, Stu Cohen, Alan Donelson, William Evans, James Hedlund, Susan Partyka, and David Skinner. I would like to thank each of the participants for their contributions, even though it is not possible to identify their personal ideas.

Financial support for the conference and book was graciously provided by the U.S. Centers for Disease Control in the form of a grant to NEIPRC. I owe special thanks to Stuart Brown of CDC and Bernard Guyer of NEIPRC for their support and encouragement. Some of the literature review contained in Chapter 1 was supported by the Motor Vehicle Manufacturers Association. In this regard, I thank Lester Lave, Henry Piehler, and Larry Slimak for their support and comments. Conference management was performed with competence and a touch of warm hospitality by Ruth Rappaport of the Educational Development Center. Thanks are also due to Dana Gelb, Doreen Neville, and Michelle Orza for conducting necessary literature reviews prior to the conference.

JOHN D. GRAHAM

March 1988   *Harvard School of Public Health*
Boston, Massachusetts

19196

CONTENTS

THE CONTRIBUTORS

Stuart T. Brown, M.D., is director, Injury Epidemiology and Control Division, Center for Environmental Health and Injury Control of the Centers for Disease Control (CDC). His principal interest is the development of a national injury control field which reflects a breadth of expertise in clinical care, engineering, and public health, and leads to reductions in morbidity, mortality, and disabilities resulting from injury. He has worked with CDC for 15 years in city/county public health programs in a clinical research and training role. He has had assignments with the World Health Organization and other international entities and has worked in other broadly based staff and management positions.

B. J. Campbell, Ph.D., is director of the University of North Carolina Highway Safety Research Center, and is a research professor of psychology. His principal research interests include automobile crash research with emphasis on program evaluation and vehicle crashworthiness.

Frances A. Campbell, Ph.D., received her degree in clinical psychology from the University of North Carolina at Chapel Hill where she is Coordinator of Psychoeducational Services, Frank Porter Graham Child Development Center. At present she is involved in a long-term study of the effects of early intervention on a group of children deemed at high risk for mild mental retardation. She has also collaborated, at times, in research on motor vehicle crashes.

Philip J. Cook, Ph.D., is professor of public policy and economics at Duke University. He has served as director of the Duke Institute of Policy Sciences since 1985. His principal research interests include the economics of unhealthy, unsafe, and imprudent behavior; the preventive effects of punishment for crime; and violent crime (with focus on the role of weapons). He has recently completed a study of robbery violence, and is currently completing an edited volume on "Vice." Currently his main research focus is the state lotteries.

Leonard Evans is a principal research scientist in the Operating Sciences Department of General Motors Research Laboratories. He has a B.Sc. degree in physics from the Queen's University of Belfast, and a D.Phil. degree in physics from Oxford University. Dr. Evans's more than 70 technical publications cover such diverse subjects as physics, mathematics, traffic engineering, transportation energy, human factors, trauma analysis, and traffic safety. His main professional interests focus on traffic safety research.

Barry Felrice is associate administrator for rulemaking of the National Highway Traffic Safety Administration of the U.S. Department of Transportation. He is the principal advisor to the administrator on all matters relating to setting and amending motor vehicle safety standards. He has been with DOT for 19 years and has a Bachelor's and Master's degree in civil engineering.

Steven Garber, Ph.D., is associate professor of economics at the School of Urban and Public Affairs at Carnegie-Mellon University. Much of his research applies microeconomic and statistical theory to public policy issues. He is particularly enthusiastic about interdisciplinary research, and past work draws on literatures in engineering, political science, psychology, and sociology, as well as economics and statistics. Past research has considered income maintenance, defense procurement, energy policy, antitrust policy, criminal sentencing, automobile safety, and coal mine safety. His current research focus is the political economy of public utility regulation, with emphasis on state regulation of telecommunications.

John D. Graham, Ph.D., is associate professor of policy and decision sciences at the Harvard School of Public Health, and deputy director of the New England Injury Prevention Research Center. His principal research interests include AIDS and public policy, environmental health regulation, and prevention of motor vehicle injuries. He is the author of two forthcoming books: *In Search of Safety: Chemicals and Cancer Risk* (1988), and *Auto Safety Through Pluralism* (1989).

Michael Grossman, Ph.D., is professor of economics at the City University of New York Graduate School and research associate and co-program director of Health Economics Research at the National Bureau of Economic Research. His principal research interests include economic models of the determinants of health, public policy, and infant mortality in the United States, and the effects of prices, excise taxes, and other regulatory variables on alcohol consumption, motor vehicle accident mortality, and cigarette smoking. He published two papers on youth motor vehicle fatalities in 1987 with Henry Saffer: "Beer Taxes, the Legal Drinking

Age, and Youth Motor Vehicle Fatalities" (*Journal of Legal Studies,* June 1987) and "Drinking Age Laws and Highway Mortality Rates: Cause and Effect" (*Economic Inquiry,* July 1987). His paper with Douglas Coate entitled "Effects of Alcohol Beverage Prices and Legal Drinking Ages on Youth Alcohol Use" appeared in the *Journal of Law and Economics* in April 1988.

Frank A. Haight, Ph.D., is adjunct professor at the Institute of Transportation Studies, University of California, Irvine. He has conducted research in mathematics and probability, and transportation and queuing theory, and, in addition, has published about 35 papers in various aspects of traffic safety. His published books include *Mathematical Theories of Traffic Flow* (Academic Press, 1963), *Handbook of the Poisson Distribution* (John Wiley, 1967), and *Applied Probability* (Plenum, 1981).

Max Henrion is an assistant professor at Carnegie-Mellon University with a joint appointment in the Department of Engineering and Public Policy and the Department of Social and Decision Sciences. He teaches decision analysis and decision support systems. He has an M.A. in psychology and statistics from the University of Cambridge (England) and a Master of Design degree from the Royal College of Art in London. His Ph.D. is in Decision Theory from the Carnegie-Mellon School of Urban and Public Affairs. A primary theme of his research has been the study of uncertainty including the psychology of how people make adjustments under uncertainty, the use of Bayesian decision theory as a guide to how one ought to reason under uncertainty, and the development of computer aids to make this more practical. He has published over 20 articles on the theory and practice of coping with uncertainty. In recent work he has been comparing decision analysis and artificial intelligence approaches to uncertain reasoning, and is exploring these two competitive paradigms in the hope of developing a synthesis.

Ralph Hingson, Sc.D., is professor and chief of Social and Behavioral Sciences at the Boston University School of Public Health and co-principal investigator of the New England Injury Prevention Research Center. His principal areas of research include injury prevention, traffic safety, alcohol and substance abuse treatment and prevention, and AIDS education evaluation.

Harold D. Holder is director of the Prevention Research Center, Berkeley, California, a national research center sponsored by the National Institute on Alcohol Abuse and Alcoholism. Dr. Holder has undertaken a number of research projects including the application of computer simulation to community planning for alcohol problem prevention, the effects of changes in distilled spirits availability on drinking levels and traffic safety, and health care costs and costs-savings associated with alcoholism treatment. He is the editor of a 1987 book entitled, *Control Issues in Alcohol Abuse Prevention: Strategies for States and Communities*, JAI Press.

Jonathan Howland, Ph.D., is an assistant professor of public health at the School of Public Health, Boston University School of Medicine. His current areas of research include predicting health services utilization using physiologic and behavioral chronic disease risk factors and injury epidemiology. He has published a number of literature reviews on the role of drinking in specific kinds of unintentional injuries (e.g., falls, fire and burn injuries, drownings).

Dana B. Kamerud, Ph.D., is senior research scientist in the Operating Sciences Department at General Motors Research Laboratories. His research interests include traffic safety, risk analysis, auto theft, and marketing research techniques. He is the author of recent articles in *Risk Analysis* and the *Journal of Policy Analysis and Management*.

Eric Latimer, M.S., is Ph.D. candidate in economics at Carnegie-Mellon University. His doctoral thesis deals with the political economy and the effectiveness of safety belt legislation in the United States.

Lester B. Lave is James H. Higgins Professor of Economics at the Graduate School of Industrial Administration at Carnegie-Mellon University, with appointments in the Department of Engineering and Public Policy and the School of Urban and Public Affairs. His research has focused on risk analysis and management, including air pollution, the identification and management of potentially toxic chemicals, public health, and the safety of dams, among other subjects. He is the co-author (with R. Crandall, H. Gruenspecht, and T. Keller) of *Regulating the Automobile*, Washington: Brookings, 1986; (with E. Latimer) "Initial Effects of the New York State Auto Safety Belt Law," *American Journal of Public Health*, 77, 183–6, 1987; "Injury as Externality: An Economic Perspective of Trauma," *Accident Analysis and Prevention*, 19, 29–37, 1987; "Health and Safety Risk Analysis: Information for Better Decisions," *Science*, 236, 291–5, 1987.

Adrian K. Lund, Ph.D., is Director of Human and Environmental Factors Research with the Insurance Institute for Highway Safety, Washington, D.C. He holds a Ph.D. in social psychology from State University of New York at Buffalo. Dr. Lund's general research interests are in the area of health behavior and the role of the individual in public health. He has researched several areas of driver behavior including risk taking, seat belt use, alcohol-impaired driving and post licensure driver training.

Brian O'Neill is president of the Insurance Institute for Highway Safety (IIHS) and its associated organization, the Highway Loss Data Institute (HLDI). These independent research and communications organizations, which are supported by U.S. property and casualty insurers, identify and develop ways to reduce the deaths, injuries, and property damage resulting from motor vehicle crashes. Mr. O'Neill, who previously served as IIHS vice president for research, has been involved in research covering all aspects of highway loss reduction, including vehicle and highway design, emergency medical care, the effectiveness of traffic laws, and driver behavior. He is author of numerous scientific papers and co-author of *The Injury Fact Book* (1984). He has served on numerous groups including the Department of Transportation's Motor Vehicle Safety Research Advisory Committee, National Accident Sampling System Advisory Committee, the National Academy of Sciences Committees on Trauma Research, and Geometric Design Standards for Highway Improvements.

Charles E. Phelps, Ph.D., is professor of political science and economics at the University of Rochester. He also directs the Public Policy Analysis Program at the University. He is co-editor of the *Journal of Policy Analysis and Management.* His principal research includes health care policy, regulation, energy policy, and natural resources policy. Recent published papers include two studies of drunk driving in youths. He is also active in studies to evaluate the use of medical diagnostic devices. Before coming to the University of Rochester in 1984, Phelps was director of the Regulatory Policies and Institutions Program, and senior economist at the Rand Corporation, Santa Monica, California.

H. Laurence Ross, Ph.D., is professor of sociology at the University of New Mexico. He has written extensively on the sociology of law, with a particular interest in the capabilities and limitations of law as a tool of behavior change. His major work in this area is *Deterring the Drinking Driver: Legal Policy and Social Control* (1982; 2nd ed., 1984). He is a member of the International Committee on Alcohol, Drugs and Traffic Safety, and serves on committees of the National Safety Council and the Transportation Research Board of the National Academy of Sciences.

Herb M. Simpson, Ph.D., is executive director of the Traffic Injury Research Foundation of Canada, a non-profit, independent research institute. His principal research interests include alcohol, drugs, and traffic safety; young driver accidents, elderly road users, occupant restraint systems, driver licensing, and improvement programs; and the evaluation of countermeasures. He is author or co-author of over 60 reports and articles on traffic safety and has served as a consultant to government and industry in many countries.

Judith Lee Stone has served as executive director of the National Association of Governors' Highway Safety Representatives (NAGHSR) since April 1982. Before joining NAGHSR, she worked for four years during the Carter Administration at the U.S. Department of Transportation, first for National Highway Traffic Safety Administrator Joan Claybrook as her special assistant and congressional relations officer, and then as director of the Secretary's Office of Consumer Liaison. As NAGHSR executive director she has written and spoken on highway safety issues such as impaired driving, occupant protection, and speed, particularly as they relate to state highway safety program management and leadership.

John Versace, Ph.D., is executive engineer for safety research in Ford Motor Company's Environmental and Safety Engineering staff. Under his direction, investigations are carried out in impact dynamics, human factors, and accident data. He is a fellow of both the American Psychological Association and the Society of Automotive Engineers.

Robert B. Voas, Ph.D., is president of Pyramid Planning, a research and development company specializing in alcohol safety and highway safety programs. His principal interests include the formulation and the evaluation of public policy and programs in the drinking driving field, and the development and application of new alcohol sensing technology. He is the author of a chapter on "Emerging Technologies for Controlling the Drunk Driver" in a book *(The Social Control of Drinking and Driving)*, published by the University of Chicago Press in January 1988.

Alexander C. Wagenaar, Ph.D., is an associate research scientist at the University of Michigan, with appointments at both the Transportation Research Institute and the School of Public Health. He is the author of *Alcohol, Young Drivers, and Traffic Accidents*, published by D. C. Heath and Company in 1983. His articles on highway safety, alcohol policy, and injury prevention have appeared in the *Journal of Trauma, Journal of Safety Research, Accident Analysis and Prevention, Pediatrics, Public Health Reports, Journal of Studies on Alcohol, British Journal of Addiction, International Journal of Addictions, Contemporary Drug Problems*, and *Journal of Public Health Policy*. Dr. Wagenaar is active in several professional organizations and currently serves on the Governing Council of the American Public Health Association.

Allan F. Williams is vice president for research of the Insurance

Institute for Highway Safety (IIHS). Prior to becoming vice president for research, Dr. Williams was senior behavioral scientist at IIHS. He has been involved in a wide variety of research areas, including alcohol, drugs and driving; seat belt use; and preventing motor vehicle deaths and injuries among teenagers and children. Before joining the Institute in 1972, Dr. Williams was project director at the Medical Foundation, Inc., Boston, Massachusetts, and a research analyst at the Massachusetts Department of Public Health. He has authored more than 100 scientific papers in professional journals. Dr. Williams received a B.A. in Psychology from Wesleyan University in 1961, and a Ph.D. in social psychology from Harvard University in 1965.

Chapter 1

INJURY CONTROL, TRAFFIC SAFETY, AND EVALUATION RESEARCH

by John D. Graham

In 1985 the Institute of Medicine (IOM) of the National Academy of Sciences commissioned a panel of experts to define the problem of "injury" in America, to assess the magnitude of the problem, and to recommend a research strategy for the nation. The panel concluded that injuries—unintentional and intentional—are the leading cause of death and disability in children and young adults. They are responsible each year for 140,000 premature deaths, 80,000 cases of permanently disabling brain and spinal cord damage, millions of visits to hospital emergency rooms, and $75 to $100 billion in direct and indirect costs to society (IOM, 1985).

The IOM panel also assessed the nation's commitment to basic and applied research about injury. Panel members concluded that research efforts on injury are "unfocused, lack continuity, and are undersupported." To help remedy this problem, the panel recommended the establishment of a new center on injury control within the Centers for Disease Control (CDC) of the Department of Health and Human Services. The panel also recommended that federal funding for injury control research be substantially increased.

In response to the concerted efforts of Congressman William Lehman (D-Fla.) and other injury control advocates, a start has been made to implement the IOM's recommendations. A new

1

Division of Injury Epidemiology and Control has been created within the Centers for Disease Control, and five academic centers of excellence have been launched across the country. Other federal agencies and several private foundations are beginning to support injury-related research and demonstration programs. Regardless of the longevity of the small CDC-related efforts, it is clear that injury is slowly becoming recognized as a major public health problem that requires serious attention.

This book relates the emerging interest in injury control to two fields of scholarly research: the science of traffic safety and quantitative methods of program evaluation. The central premise of the book is that injury control, while currently dominated by political advocacy, can gain greater credibility by developing analytical linkages to these established fields of scientific inquiry. In this introductory chapter, the reader is offered a broad overview of the science of traffic safety and state-of-the-art approaches to evaluating traffic injury countermeasures.

Dimensions of the Problem

The largest single cause of injury in America is the motor vehicle crash. In 1986 such crashes were responsible for 46,000 fatalities, 3.4 million disabling injuries, and a majority of the direct and indirect costs of injury to society. At current crash-injury rates, about one in every 70 persons born this year will ultimately die in a crash. The corresponding lifetime risk of disabling injury from crashes is one in three.

Since everyone must die sooner or later of some cause, it is useful to also consider various measures of premature death. While motor vehicle crashes are the seventh leading cause of death, they are also the third leading cause of "early death," defined as death before age 65. Only cancer and heart disease are responsible for a larger number of early deaths. Crash-related injuries are also the third leading cause of life years lost, again following cancer and heart disease. The key point is that motor vehicle injuries strike primarily the young. The average crash victim is 34 years old. Among Americans between the ages of 1 and 40, motor vehicle injuries are the number one cause of death.

The vast majority of crash-related injuries have no permanent adverse effect on a motorist's physical or mental health. The most frequent types of injuries are bruises, lacerations, and simple fractures of the motorist's extremities. Medical care and time can repair most of these problems, thereby allowing people to resume normal lives. Some types of injuries, however, are less likely to be repaired and instead result in lifelong impairment. In particular, injuries to a motorist's skull, face, or spinal cord have troublesome prognoses. In severe cases these injuries can result in conditions such as brain damage, epilepsy, blindness, paraplegia, or quadra-plegia. While it is known that crashes are a major cause of these impairments, there is no national data system that records the incidence of permanent impairments resulting from crashes. More comprehensive studies of the incidence and costs of nonfatal crash injuries are now underway under the joint sponsorship of the U.S. Department of Transportation and CDC.

Trends in Crash-Related Mortality

Since World War II, the total number of crash-related deaths has increased substantially, from 28,100 in 1945 to a peak of 56,300 in 1972. The energy crisis and adoption of the maximum 55 mph speed limit caused a sharp drop in the death toll to 46,400 in 1974. Yet the toll resumed its upward trend throughout the remainder of the 1970s until it reached 53,000 in 1979. Then the severe reces-sion of 1981–1983 and renewed attention to drunk driving counter-measures helped reduce the toll to 44,600 in 1983. In recent years a modest upward trend in traffic deaths has accompanied the return of economic prosperity.

The postwar period witnessed a large growth in population and affluence. These factors in turn caused large increases in the number of motor vehicles, the number of licensed drivers, and the number of vehicle miles traveled (VMT). For a different historical perspective, it is useful to examine trends in motor vehicle death *rates*, measured as the number of deaths per 100 million VMT and the number of deaths per 100,000 population. Figure 1–1 displays trends in these rates for the period 1947–1984.

The death rate per mile has—except for only a few years—been declining since World War II. Death counts have increased because the growth in travel has simply outpaced the fall in the death rate per mile. Causes of the decline in the mileage death rate are not well understood, but the following explanations have been offered: (1) a suspected decline in the number of occupants per vehicle, possibly reflecting growth in the ratio of vehicles to population; (2) a shift from rural to safer urban travel instigated by urbanization of the American economy; and (3) some combination of safer vehicles, better educated drivers, and better designed roads, especially completion of the interstate highway system.

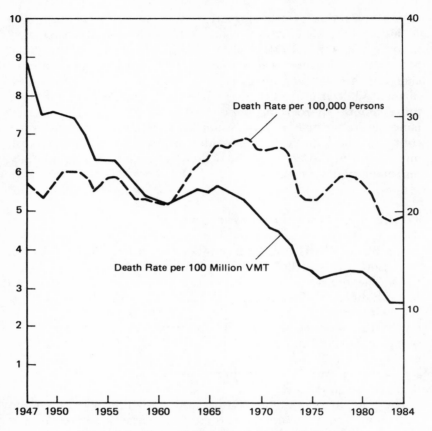

Figure 1-1   Motor Vehicle Death Rates, 1947-1984.

Public health specialists are more inclined to express motor
vehicle death rates on a population basis, the method used to
express rates of death from other causes. When measured with
this yardstick, the historical trends are not so favorable (see Figure
1–1). In the 1950s, the death rate was roughly flat but then
increased to a peak of 27.6 per 100,000 persons in 1969. After the
sharp drop in 1974, the rate was roughly constant until another
dip down during the 1981–1983 recession. When viewed over the
entire postwar period, the population death rate has been remark-
ably stable. Apparently, the favorable trends in driver performance, vehicle design, and highway safety have been continually
offset by increases in travel and other unfavorable factors. Overall,
the population death rate from crashes was only about 12 percent
lower in 1984 than it was in 1947.

Additional insight into historical patterns is gained by disaggregating the death toll by vehicle type. Such a breakdown is presented in Figure 1–2 for 1965–1983, the time period for which such data are available. As a fraction of total deaths, occupants of passenger cars have declined from two-thirds to almost one-half. The contribution of pedestrians has been roughly flat. The diminishing relative significance of automobiles is accompanied by the rising significance of trucks and two-wheeled vehicles (motorcycles and bicycles). This breakdown of the problem is informative because it suggests that injury controllers should consider placing somewhat more emphasis on trucks and two-wheeled vehicles relative to passenger cars.

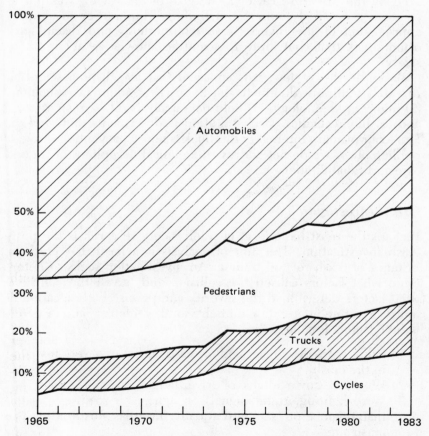

Figure 1-2   Percentage of Motor Vehicle Fatalities by Vehicle Type, 1965–1983.

Research Traditions in Traffic Safety

Compared to other causes of injuries, motor vehicle crashes have already been studied extensively. In order to characterize the major research traditions that have contributed to knowledge about traffic safety, we undertook a comprehensive review of articles published since 1980. This review encompasses articles in peer-reviewed scientific journals and articles published by the Society for Automotive Engineers (SAE). Telephone interviews with selected researchers in the motor vehicle industry, the federal government, and academic and nonprofit research institutions supplemented the literature review. Often these interviews called attention to additional articles of importance that were not uncovered by the literature review. The goal of the review was not to produce a detailed summary of findings, but rather to gain an appreciation of the diverse research methods and disciplinary orientations that contribute to scientific knowledge about traffic safety.

Based on this review, it is apparent that five distinct scientific research traditions dominate the field: (1) accident investigation, (2) injury epidemiology, (3) field data analysis, (4) human factors, and (5) biomechanics. Each tradition is described briefly below. Since our primary interest in this book is injury prevention through public policy, we do not address the clinical disciplines of trauma care and rehabilitation.

Crash Investigation

Perhaps the most basic form of traffic safety research is the post-crash investigation. The unit of analysis is a particular crash or instance of crash-related trauma. An investigation seeks to determine what factors caused the collision and, given the collision, what factors determined the severity and precise body location of injury. Routine information on behavioral, vehicular, and environmental factors is collected:

1. What types of vehicles and/or roadside fixtures were involved in the crash?
2. Was there any evidence of driver fatigue or inebriation?
3. Were lighting, traffic signals or signs, and roadway design/maintenance of "standard" quality in areas surrounding the crash site?
4. Was there any evidence of vehicular defects such as brake failure or tire blowout?

Answers to these questions might lead an investigator to develop an opinion about the proximate, primary, and secondary causes of the collision.

Given the collision, a medical examiner may survey the condition of the injured occupant(s) and the vehicle(s). Basic descriptive information might include:

1. What body locations suffered injury?
2. Was the occupant ejected from the passenger compartment and, if so, what were the ultimate physical sources of body impact?
3. If the occupant remained in the passenger compartment, was there any external source of intrusion into the passenger compartment that contributed to injury?
4. If the passenger compartment remained intact, which surfaces or objects in the vehicle interior made contact with the occupant during the "second collision"?

Where available, information on occupant belt use and the occupant's age and medical condition may also be collected. Using all of the above information, the investigator may develop an informed opinion about how the severity of injury (given the collision) could have been mitigated.

Details about a particular crash are not normally of scientific interest because a single crash situation cannot be generalized. Not surprisingly, only a tiny proportion of crash investigations result in some scientific publication. Those that do tend to involve highly unusual events. For example, the recent medical literature contains case reports on whiplash injuries induced by safety belts (Clarke and Whittaker, 1981; Denis et al., 1983), injuries caused by motorcycle helmets (Walsh and Trotter, 1979–1980), and fatal injury to bicyclists from rearview car windows (Fife et al., 1983). Lack of publication does not mean that crash investigators do not collect scientific knowledge about traffic safety. Professional crash investigators learn about the details of hundreds of crashes during their career. While their samples are not necessarily random, their cumulative understanding of real-world crash environments is rich and sophisticated. Thus, injury controllers must devise techniques to elicit the expertise of crash investigators who may have little incentive or inclination to publish their "findings."

Injury Epidemiology

Epidemiologists are concerned with documenting the incidence of crash-related injury and discovering systematic patterns in the incidence of injury. Sources of data may include hospital records, police reports, coroners' reports, or findings from special crash investigations. Since nationwide epidemiological studies are too expensive, the researcher will typically focus on a particular jurisdiction or geographical location for which high-quality data are available or can be readily collected.

To a large extent injury epidemiology is a descriptive enterprise. The following types of questions might be addressed:

1. How does the rate of pedestrian (occupant) injury vary by age of the pedestrian (occupant)?
2. How many cases of spinal cord injury are caused each year by motor vehicle crashes?
3. In what proportion of fatal and nonfatal crashes is the driver known to be intoxicated by drugs or alcohol?

Answers to these questions do not necessarily have decisive implications for the design or efficacy of countermeasures. They may, however, point to problems or patterns of injury that deserve more attention by injury controllers.

Major efforts have been made to document the incidence of permanent health impairments resulting from crash-related injuries. Such studies have shown that crashes are a frequent cause of spinal cord injury (Smart and Sanders, 1976), brain damage (Kraus et al., 1984), facial fractures (Karlson, 1982), epilepsy (CCEC, 1978), and blindness (Huelke, O'Day, and Barhydt, 1982). Other studies show that lower extremity and chest injuries from crashes are more prevalent and medically serious than previously thought (Huelke, O'Day, and Barhydt, 1982; Newman and Jones, 1984; Newman and Rastogi, 1984). These studies are not necessarily useful for purposes of identifying countermeasures, but they serve the purpose of documenting the seriousness of the injury problem.

Field Data Analysis

This research tradition uses historical data on crashes and injury to understand the traffic safety system. The analyst's challenge is to isolate and quantify the influences of various independent variables such as driver attributes, vehicle characteristics, and environmental conditions. The disciplinary backgrounds of such analysts are quite diverse, but there is a shared conviction that multivariate statistical methods can be fruitfully employed to gain knowledge about the injury problem.

For decades this research strategy was plagued by severe data deficiencies. Traditional sources of crash and injury data were the

National Safety Council and state transportation departments (NSC, 1984). Reported data on fatalities from these sources are fairly reliable, but variation in police reporting practices among localities makes the collision and nonfatal injury data somewhat suspect and inconsistent. More importantly, these sources report relatively little reliable information on the primary independent variables of interest: drivers, vehicles, and environmental conditions.

While many data limitations remain, progress has been made in recent years. The National Highway Traffic Safety Administration (NHTSA) has created several new national data bases. The Fatal Accident Reporting System (FARS) is a computerized system with detailed information on every motor vehicle fatality that has occurred in the United States since 1975 (FARS, 1983). The National Accident Sampling System (NASS) was created in 1979 to provide a representative sample of all police-reported crashes in the United States. Research teams at 75 NASS sites throughout the country report detailed information on about 15,000 crashes each year (NASS, 1981). Finally, the National Crash Severity Study (NCSS) was an investigation of 7,000 automobile crashes that occurred in seven urban areas of the United States from January 1977 to March 1979. Detailed information is available on velocity prior to impact, extent of vehicle damage, and types of occupant injuries (Ricci, 1979). These new data systems, especially FARS, have stimulated a virtual explosion in the number of statistical studies of the traffic safety system.

One stream of research seeks to understand the quantitative relationship between driver characteristics and collision frequency and injury severity. For instance, researchers have established the importance of human factors such as age of driver, speed of vehicle, prior accident record of driver, safety belt use, and type of optical lens worn by the driver. A parallel stream of research investigates the role of vehicle attributes such as age of vehicle, type of belt design, fuel tank design, size or weight of vehicle, roof design, and the presence of rear-mounted brake lights. A third stream of research focuses on the role of environmental conditions such as weather, traffic density, road type, time of day or week, and prevailing business conditions. The more sophisticated studies attempt to measure simultaneously the effects of various driver, vehicle, and environmental variables.

Human Factors

A large literature in traffic safety addresses the role of human behavior in causing collisions and injury. One stream of studies seeks to measure "risky" driving and predict such behavior using demographic, vehicular, and law enforcement data. A different stream of work seeks to determine the potential and actual performance of humans in executing driving tasks in various situations. Both lines of inquiry rely on three sources of behavioral data: testing of subjects on driving simulators; observation of volunteer subjects in the field (possibly with the aid of an instrumented car); and direct observation of the real-world driving behavior of unsuspecting motorists.

Several indicators of risky driving behavior have been proposed. These include following distance, acceptance gaps, vehicle speed, lane keeping, time headway, and driver reactions to stop or yield signs. These measures are then used as dependent variables in analyses of the determinants of risky driving behavior. Special attention has been given to comparing the driving behavior of those with crash histories to those with no such histories. Unfortunately, this stream of research offers no direct insights about countermeasures, although the measures of risk taking are useful for testing theories of behavioral response to countermeasures.

The other line of inquiry seeks to define the limits of human driving capabilities and devise educational methods that permit drivers to fulfill these capabilities. Where driving situations entail performance of tasks in excess of human capability, alterations in roads and/or vehicles may be appropriate. The driving task is complicated by numerous factors, and investigators are trying to understand the impact of such complications on driver behavior. Recent studies have addressed issues such as the influence of fatigue on driving performance, driver response times to traffic signals under various conditions, the influence of moderate alcohol intake on driving performance, and driver reactions to freeway construction zones and to vehicles with high-mounted rear brake lights.

Driver vision is a key concept in human factors research, but vision research is complicated by the interaction of vision competence with human motivation. For example, much attention has been given to the problem of impaired driver vision during nighttime travel. But one interesting study found that poor ability to see traffic signs at night was more than compensated for by higher levels of driver attention and care at night. The motivational effect can also work to the detriment of safety. The presence of stop signs at intersections, for instance, may sometimes reduce driver caution when making turns. Other issues where vision plays a key role include rural curve negotiation, driver perception of pedestrians at night, the conspicuity of motorcycles with and without daytime headlights, the problem of glare from vehicle headlamps and headlights, and the effect of bad weather on driver seeing distance.

Investigators also examine the speed of driver reaction to various exogenous events, because reaction time is believed to be important in crash avoidance. Response time to events varies among drivers and situations, especially when the driver's attention is distracted by other tasks. Events that have been the subject of response-time studies include the opening of parked car doors in front of traffic, abrupt-onset cross winds, presence of left and right directional signs, and oncoming vehicles near the center line of a two-lane road.

In addition to drivers, the behavior of pedestrians and vehicle passengers are important topics in human factors research. Child road-crossing behavior has been the subject of recent study. Apparently, progress is being made in devising educational programs that induce children to cross streets more safely. The dominant issue in passenger safety is clearly adult and infant restraint use. The burgeoning literature on this topic examines belt use as a function of demographics, attitudes, incentives, education, legislation, and police enforcement. The topic has received more interest in the United States recently due to the trend toward passage of compulsory belt use laws by state legislatures.

Biomechanics

The field of biomechanics has a rich research tradition related to both human injury resulting from collisions and laboratory studies and performance tests on human surrogates. Biomechanics encompasses many areas of investigation not germane to automobile collisions—for example, the rheology of blood flow and the dynamics of the human gait. However, the biomechanics of impacts is absolutely essential to analyze the origins of crash-related injury and the effectiveness of potential injury-reducing strategies.

Research on the biomechanics of impacts can be characterized according to emphasis on specific regions of the body: the musculoskeletal system, the head and neck, the thorax, the abdomen, the pelvis, the extremities, and the nervous system.

Inspired performance testing to characterize the crashworthiness of vehicles has caused research efforts to be focused in the following areas of concern: (1) knowledge of crash forces, accelerations, or displacements and their time histories; (2) knowledge of human tolerance to these forces and displacements; (3) availability of surrogates, either physical or mathematical, to study and evaluate responses to crash-related forces; and (4) knowledge of the distributions of real-world collisions by source of impact (e.g., frontal vs. lateral vs. rear-end collisions). These performance-based characterizations can be augmented with concepts developed by Rowe (1983) to produce several other functionally based subdivisions of impact-related biomechanics research. These include: (1) selecting and obtaining results from performance tests on human surrogates (e.g., specific tests and results of tests on dummies, cadavers, and animals); (2) internal validation of tests on surrogates (e.g., repeatability and reproducibility of tests on surrogates, comparisons of test results among different types of surrogates, plus evaluations of the effects of different conditions of individual surrogates on performance-test results); (3) performing case studies to characterize injury in actual crashes; (4) internal validation of the techniques and indices used to quantify trauma in actual crashes; (5) development of translational models that link the results of performance tests on surrogates to injury experienced in actual crashes; and (6) the internal validation of these translational models that link performance-test results to injury experienced in actual crashes.

*   *   *

By describing biomechanics and the other research areas as distinct traditions, one might surmise that participating scientists work in total isolation from one another. To the contrary, the research traditions come together at a variety of multidisciplinary research organizations such as the Insurance Institute for Highway Safety, the General Motors Research Laboratories, the University of North Carolina Highway Safety Research Center, the University of Michigan Transportation Research Institute, and the National Highway Traffic Safety Administration. And, as we shall describe below, the ultimate challenge is to bring the traditions together when devising injury control policies.

Countermeasure Development and Evaluation

In order to translate scientific knowledge about crash-related injury into a real-world reduction in the incidence of injury, effective countermeasures (or "interventions") must be devised and implemented. To clarify thinking about countermeasure development, William Haddon, Jr., M.D., devised in the early 1960s a conceptual scheme to describe intervention opportunities. The so-called "Haddon matrix," which is reprinted in Figure 1–3, postulates that human, vehicular, and environmental factors operate

Factors

Phases	Human	Vehicles and Equipment	Physical and Socio-economic Environment
Pre-crash			
Crash			
Post-crash			

Losses	Damage to People	Damage to Vehicles and Equipment	Damage to Physical and Socio-economic Environment

Figure 1-3   The Haddon Matrix.

during the precrash, crash, and postcrash phases to produce injuries. The challenge for professional injury controllers is to use scientific knowledge to discover the most effective (and cost-effective) countermeasures within each cell of the matrix.

The research traditions described above have played a critical role in stimulating countermeasure development. Crash investigators, epidemiologists, statisticians, and human factors specialists have, for example, pinpointed alcohol as a causative factor in many motor vehicle crashes. This research has in turn provided a scientific basis for a variety of drunk driving countermeasures. Likewise, biomechanics research and field data analysis have highlighted the importance of occupant restraint systems and vehicle speed in determining the severity of crash injury. Hence, we observe careful consideration of occupant-restraint policy and highway speed limits.

A scientific consensus already exists that countermeasures can be devised to diminish the contribution of (at least) three injury-enhancing factors: driver inebriation, nonuse of occupant restraints, and excessive vehicle speed. Despite this consensus, the precise implications for development of the countermeasure is not clear. The missing information needs to be provided by what might be called "evaluation research": quantitative estimates of the consequences (safety and nonsafety) of decision alternatives that are faced by public and private decision makers.

The need for reliable evaluation research is becoming increasingly important as the public begins to recognize the injury problem and to demand adoption of countermeasures. The last decade in particular has been a period of remarkable change in traffic safety policy. In the early 1980s grass-roots activists such as Mothers Against Drunk Driving (MADD) spawned a nationwide effort to punish and curtail drunken driving. Numerous reforms of drunk driving laws have been enacted. Simultaneously, many states in the country were enacting laws that require parents to restrain their young children during motor vehicle travel. The occupant-restraint movement then spread to adults as state after state passed laws compelling all motorists to wear manual safety belts. In response to federal regulation, car manufacturers are also beginning to offer innovative automatic belt systems and improved air bag designs.

· The recent policy changes have not been all in the direction of more safety. In particular, Congress has recently withdrawn the authority of the federal government to withhold highway funds from states that fail to enforce the national maximum 55 mph speed limit. In many states the maximum speed limits on rural interstates have been raised to 65 mph. Similar speed limit reforms may soon be applied to many noninterstate rural highways.

The principal challenge for the evaluation research community is to assess accurately the beneficial and adverse consequences of these policy reforms. This book presents state-of-the-art evaluation methods and up-to-date findings on these three classes of injury control policies. Some of the methods employed are retrospective (i.e., evaluation of past policies), while others are prospective (i.e., evaluation of future policy scenarios). The findings of evaluation research, to the extent they are trustworthy, should be helpful to injury control advocates and policymakers as they set their own agendas for the 1990s. The purpose of evaluation research is therefore to build an analytical bridge between scientific investigation of injury and advocacy of injury control interventions.

Since evaluation is a bridge between science and policy, it should not be surprising that there are no value-free evaluation studies. A value framework is implicit or explicit in the evaluation of any injury control intervention. By their very nature, choices about what to evaluate and which outcomes to measure are value-laden.

The two most common value frameworks used in traffic safety evaluation might be called "the public health ethic" and the "cost-benefit ethic." Public health advocates argue that the best injury control interventions are those that promise the largest absolute reduction in the incidence (or severity) of injury. While this approach confronts some subsidiary value judgments about the relative importance of various types of injuries, the outcome measures are based exclusively on injury information. In contrast, the cost-benefit analyst seeks adoption of those injury control policies that maximize the difference between the incremental dollar benefits and costs of intervention. The overriding metric is economic, and all policy consequences (to the extent possible) are converted to a monetary metric. The opportunity for policy consensus among evaluators is greatest for those countermeasures that pass both the public health and benefit-cost tests.

The Mechanics of Evaluation Research

Although evaluation research is often difficult and controversial, the process can be explained simply. An evaluation entails four steps: (1) selection of countermeasures to be studied, (2) selection of outcome measures, (3) data collection, and (4) selection of analytic methods and their application to available data. Important judgments must be made at each step.

The selection of countermeasures for study cannot be performed in a strictly scientific fashion. There are an infinite number of countermeasures that could be considered in an evaluation, and it is difficult to justify (scientifically) restrictions on the number or types of countermeasures to be considered. In most evaluation studies the interventions considered are dictated by the specific legal or political context or are specified (more or less) arbitrarily by the analyst. When countermeasures are evaluated, it is nonetheless critical to specify the traffic safety conditions that would exist in the absence of the countermeasure of interest. The "status quo" is rarely well defined in traffic safety policy, and hence a precise baseline or comparison scenario needs to be specified for analytical purposes.

Several types of outcome measures are used in traffic safety policy evaluations. "Process" measures are those that reflect the impact of countermeasures on human, vehicular, and environmental factors (see the Haddon matrix in Figure 1–3). Examples of process measures include belt-use rates, self-reports of drunk driving, counts of cars with air bags, DWI arrests, and roadside speed measurements. "Injury-based" outcome measures are often more satisfying to policymakers. Examples include counts of fatal or disabling injuries or proportions of crashes resulting in injury of a specified degree of severity. "Economic" outcome measures are almost always expressed in dollar units and are usually intended to reflect the net economic consequence (benefits minus costs) of the countermeasure under study. The most comprehensive evaluation might include analysis of process, injury, and economic outcomes, although such ambitious studies are rarely performed.

The data collection for evaluation of injury control interventions is tedious and expensive, as is the case in most lines of empirical research. Information must be collected on both the various outcome measures and the countermeasures of interest (e.g., their date of adoption, degree of implementation, stringency of enforcement, and extent of compliance). Since such evaluations are most often performed in a nonexperimental context, information must also be collected on covariates that, if ignored, might obscure the true effect of the intervention. For example, increases in vehicle speeds due to relaxed police enforcement might conceal a beneficial effect of new belt-use laws on fatality counts. Alternatively, outcome information must be collected for time periods and/or jurisdictions unaffected by the countermeasure of interest. Throughout the data collection process, efforts must be made to assure high data quality and to recognize inherent weaknesses in data quality.

Selection of analytic methods is typically driven by the nature of the available data and the disciplinary orientation of the analyst. Most retrospective evaluations of traffic safety policies employ some form of nonexperimental statistical analysis. Time-series techniques are used to project injury counts assuming countermeasures had not been adopted. Projections are then compared to actual experience to infer the effects of countermeasures. This approach has been used to assess the efficacy of drunk-driving legislation (Hilton, 1984; Hingson et al., 1983; Ross et al., 1981–82; Ross, Klette, and McCleary, 1984); child-restraint laws (Wagenaar, 1985: Guerin and MacKinnon, 1984); mandatory belt use laws (MacKay, 1985; Jonah and Lawson, 1984); revised speed limits (NAS, 1984; Tofany, 1981; Frith and Toomath, 1982); and vehicle crash-survivability standards (Graham and Garber, 1984; Peltzman, 1975).

An alternative method is cross-sectional analysis where jurisdictions with and without a countermeasure of interest are compared (so-called "quasi-experimental" methods). Differences in crash or injury rates between jurisdictions are attributed to countermeasures, after the influences of confounding variables have been controlled statistically or by study design. Sometimes both time series and cross-sectional information are combined in the same evaluation model. Such methods have been used to assess the efficacy of motorcycle headlamp and helmet-wearing laws (Muller, 1984; Adams, 1983); alcohol enforcement policies (Colo'n and Cutter, 1983; Colo'n, 1983; Hauer, 1983; Norstrom, 1983; Votey

and Shapiro, 1983; Votey, 1984; Holder and Blose, 1983; Salzberg
and Paulsrude, 1984); vehicle inspection laws (Crain, 1980; Van
Matre and Overstreet, 1982; Loeb and Gilad, 1984); minimum
drinking-age laws (Williams et al., 1983; Colo'n, 1984; Wagenaar,
1983; Cook and Tauchen, 1984); driving curfew laws (Preusser,
Williams, Zador, and Blomberg, 1984); driver education programs
(Robertson, 1980); driver licensing restrictions (Preusser, Williams, and Lund, 1985); no-fault automobile insurance (Landes,
1982); and right-turn-on-red laws (Preusser et al., 1982; Zador,
Moshman, and Marcus, 1982).

Retrospective cost-benefit evaluation usually combines results
from quasi-experimental studies with estimates of the economic
costs of injuries to produce monetary benefit estimates for specific
countermeasures. Traffic injuries can cause significant damage to
the American economy. Economists have attempted to approximate this damage by calculating the monetary value of medical
resources devoted to the treatment and rehabilitation of crash
victims. In addition to these direct costs of injury, there are also
indirect costs attributable to the diminished economic productivity
of crash victims. Economists have attempted to approximate indirect costs by calculating the present value of foregone earnings
attributable to fatal and nonfatal crash injuries.

As an extension of injury epidemiology, some studies have made
detailed estimates of the economic impacts of permanent impairments such as spinal cord injury (Smart and Saunders, 1976) and
brain damage (Grabow, Offord, and Rieder, 1984). The government has used these studies and other data to generate nationwide
estimates of the total (direct and indirect) costs of crash-related
injury (NHTSA, 1983). Other investigators have attempted to
compare the economic impact of crash-related injury to the economic impact of diseases such as cancer and heart disease (Hartunian, Smart, and Thompson, 1980; Dean, West, and Meur, 1982).
They find, not surprisingly, that injury has especially large economic costs because crash victims are likely to be afflicted during
the prime productive years of their lives.

A different approach to measuring the potential economic benefits of injury reduction—one that is suggested by microeconomic
theory—is to estimate how much motorists and taxpayers are
willing to pay for various degrees of injury reduction, assuming
that safety behavior is unchanged. Some economists have tried to
infer willingness to pay for transport safety from personal decisions
or market choices. Such "revealed preference" studies have addressed new-car purchases (Winston and Mannering, 1984) and
belt use behavior (Blomquist, 1979; Dardis, 1983). The results are

difficult to interpret, among other reasons, because it is doubtful whether consumers and motorists have accurate perceptions of their personal probabilities of crash-related injury.

An alternative method is to survey motorists directly and ask them how much they would be willing to pay for various degrees of injury reduction. These "expressed preference" surveys have all the virtues and flaws of marketing surveys and opinion polls. Some recent surveys suggest that consumers would be willing to pay large amounts of money for reduced risks of crash-related injury (Muller and Reutzel, 1984; Jones-Lee, Hammerton, and Philips, 1985). Skepticism is warranted because people may be inclined to respond more liberally with verbal promises than they would actually commit with dollars from limited family budgets.

If the economic benefits of injury reduction could somehow be quantified reliably, then this information could be used in cost-benefit analyses of traffic safety countermeasures. Many such studies have been published in the literature. Recently, the passive-restraint standard has been addressed in several analyses (Arnould and Grabowksi, 1981; Nordhaus, 1981; Graham and Henrion, 1984), although the results are inconclusive due to uncertainty about various inputs such as usage of automatic belts, costs of various air-bag designs and the appropriate monetary value of injury reduction. Cost-benefit analysis has been applied to various other countermeasures as well, such as automobile child restraints (Main, 1985); state motor vehicle inspection laws (Thompson, 1985; Loeb and Gilad, 1984); police enforcement campaigns (Helander, 1984); the 55 mph speed limit (Jondrow, Bowes, and Levy, 1983; NAS, 1984); motorcycle helmet-wearing laws (Muller, 1980); daylight vehicle lighting policies (Attwood, 1981; Harvey, 1983); and the Pinto recall issue (Dardis and Zent, 1982).

Given the inherent uncertainty associated with cost-benefit analysis of transport safety, some analysts and decision makers prefer cost-effectiveness analysis (CEA). This technique can be used either to identify the cheapest portfolio of countermeasures that achieve a specified injury-reduction goal, or to identify the portfolio of countermeasures that avert the largest amount of injury yet do not exceed a fixed dollar budget for investment in countermeasures. Several recent studies have produced comparative cost-effectiveness estimates for a variety of behavioral, highway, and vehicular countermeasures (NHTSA, 1981; Solomon, Perkins, and Resetar, 1985).

For countermeasures that have no direct real-world experience, evaluation research is still feasible but necessarily speculative. Estimates of countermeasure effectiveness must then be based on indirect evidence of various sorts and theoretical viewpoints. Simulation and Bayesian techniques can also be used to make quantitative forecasts of the consequences of untested countermeasures, including probabilistic treatment of uncertainties. Relatively little research of this form has been published in the traffic safety literature, although two papers in this book employ these methods.

Chapters in this Volume

Each chapter in this book presents a summary of one or more pieces of evaluation research. The countermeasures include occupant restraint policy, drunk driving policy, and highway speed policy. The evaluations employ both retrospective and prospective methods, classical and Bayesian statistics, and adopt either the public health or economic framework. Each chapter is followed by commentary from several experts. Taken together, the chapters and the comments of discussants present a thorough review of the state-of-the-art methods used in traffic safety evaluation research and recent findings, including a discussion of the limitations of these methods. In the last chapter, we hazard some recommendations about scientific and policy directions for the next ten years.

References

ADAMS, J. G. U. 1983. "Public Safety Legislation and the Risk Compensation Hypothesis: The Example of Motorcycle Helmet Legislation." *Environment and Planning C: Government and Policy* 1:193–203.

ARNOULD, R. J., and H. GRABOWSKI. 1981. "Auto Safety Regulation: An Analysis of Market Failure." *Bell Journal of Economics* 12, 1:27.

ATTWOOD, D. A. 1981. "The Potential of Daytime Running Lights as a Vehicle Collision Countermeasure." SAE Technical Paper, Series No. 810190, 19 pages.

BLOMQUIST, G. 1979. "Value of Life Saving: Implications of Consumption Activity." *Journal of Political Economy* 87:541–58.

CCEC. 1978. *Plan for Nationwide Action on Epilepsy*, Staff of the Commission for the Control of Epilepsy and Its Consequences, vol. II, part 1, "Head Injury," 246.

CLARKE, P., and M. WHITTAKER. 1981. "Traumatic Aneurysm of the Internal Cartoid Artery and Rupture of the Duodenum Following Seat Belt Injury," *Injury* 12:158–60.

COLO'N, I. 1983. "County Level Prohibition and Alcohol-Related Fatal Motor Vehicle Accidents." *Journal of Safety Research* 14, 3:101.

———. 1984. "The Alcohol Beverage Purchase Age and Single Vehicle Highway Fatalities." *Journal of Safety Research* 15, 4:159.

COLO'N, I, and H. S. G. CUTTER. 1983. "The Relationship of Beer Consumption and State Alcohol and Motor Vehicle Policies to Fatal Accidents." *Journal of Safety Research* 14, no. 2:83.

COOK, P. J., and G. TAUCHEN. 1984. "The Effects of Minimum Drinking Age Legislation on Youthful Auto Fatalities." *Journal of Legal Studies* 13:169–90.

CRAIN, W. M. 1980. *Vehicle Safety Inspection Systems: How Effective?* Washington, D.C.: American Enterprise Institute.

DARDIS, R. 1983. "Consumer Risk Response and Consumer Protection: An Economic Analysis of Seat Belt Usage." *Journal of Consumer Affairs* 17:245–61.

DARDIS, R., and C. ZENT. 1982. "The Economics of the Pinto Recall." *Journal of Consumer Affairs* 16:261–77.

DEAN, A. G., D. J. WEST, and W. Z. MEUR. 1982. "Measuring Loss of Life, Health and Income due to Disease and Injury: A Method for Combining Morbidity, Mortality and Direct Medical Cost into a Single Measure of Disease Impact." *Public Health Reports* 97:38–47.

DENIS, R., M. ALLARD, H. ATLAS, and E. FARKOUH. 1983. "Changing Trends with Abdominal Injury in Seatbelt Wearers." *Journal of Trauma* 23:1007–09.

FARS. 1983. *Fatal Accident Reporting System.* U.S. Department of Transportation, National Highway Traffic Safety Administration, DOT-HS-806-251.

FIFE, D., J. DAVIS, and L. TATE. 1983. "Fatal Injuries to Bicyclists from Rear View Mirrors." *Journal of Trauma* 23:752–57.

FRITH, W. J., and J. B. TOOMATH. 1982. "The New Zealand Open Road Speed Limit." *Accident Analysis and Prevention* 14:209–18.

GRABOW, J. D., K. P. OFFORD, and M. E. RIEDER. 1984. "The Cost of Head Injury in Olmsted County, Minnesota, 1970–1974." *American Journal of Public Health* 74:710–12.

GRAHAM, J. D., and S. GARBER. 1984. "Evaluating the Effects of Automobile Safety Regulation." *Journal of Policy Analysis and Management* 3:206–24.

GRAHAM, J. D., and M. HENRION. 1984. "A Probabilistic Analysis of the Passive Restraint Question." *Risk Analysis* 4:25–41.

GUERIN, D., and D. P. MACKINNON. 1984. "An Assessment of the California Child Passenger Restraint Requirement." *American Journal of Public Health* 75:142–44.

HARTUNIAN, N. S., C. N. SMART, and M. S. THOMPSON. 1980. "The Incidence and Economic Costs of Cancer, Motor Vehicle Injuries, Coronary Heart Disease, and Stroke: A Comparative Analysis." *American Journal of Public Health* 70:1249.

HARVEY, C. M. 1983. "Cost-Benefit Study of a Proposed Daylight Running Lights Safety Programme." *Journal of the Operations Research Society* 34:37–43.

HAUER, E. 1983. "An Application of the Likelihood/Bayes Approach to the Estimation of Safety Countermeasure Effectiveness." *Accident Analysis and Prevention* 15:287–98.

HELANDER, C. J. 1984. "Intervention Strategies for Accident-Involved Drivers: An Experimental Evaluation of Current California Policy and Alternatives." *Journal of Safety Research* 15, 1:23.

HILTON, M. E. 1984. "The Impact of Recent Changes in California Drinking

Driving Laws on Fatal Accident Levels During the First Post-Intervention Year: An Interrupted Time-Series Analysis." *Law and Society Review* 18, no. 4:605.

HINGSON, R. W., et al. 1983. "Impact of Legislation Raising the Legal Drinking Age in Massachusetts from 18 to 20." *American Journal of Public Health* 73:163–70.

HOLDER, H., and J. BLOSE. 1983. "Prevention of Alcohol Related Traffic Problems: Computer Simulation of Alternative Strategies." *Journal of Safety Research* 14, 3:115.

HUELKE, D. F., J. O'DAY, and W. H. BARHYDT. 1982. "Ocular Injuries in Automobile Crashes." *Journal of Trauma* 22:50–52.

Institute of Medicine (IOM). 1985. *Injury in America*. Washington, D.C.: National Research Council.

JONAH, B. A., and J. LAWSON. 1984. "The Effectiveness of the Canadian Mandatory Seat Belt Use Laws." *Accident Analysis and Prevention* 16, no. 5–6:433–50.

JONDROW, J., M. BOWES, and R. LEVY. 1983. "The Optimal Speed Limit." *Economic Inquiry* 21:325–36.

JONES-LEE, M. W., M. HAMMERTON, and P. R. PHILIPS. 1985. "The Value of Safety: Results of a National Sample Survey." *The Economic Journal* 95:49–72.

KARLSON, T. A. "The Incidence of Hospital-Related Facial Injuries from Vehicles." *Journal of Trauma* 11:303–10.

KRAUS, J. F., et al. 1984. "The Incidence of Acute Brain Injury and Serious Impairment in a Defined Population." *American Journal of Epidemiology* 119:186.

LANDES, E. M. 1982. "Insurance, Liability, and Accidents: A Theoretical and Empirical Investigation of the Effect of No-Fault Accidents." *Journal of Law and Economics* 25:49–65.

LEWIN, I. "Driver Training: A Perceptual-Motor Skill Approach." *Ergonomics* 25:912–24.

LOEB, P., and B. GILAD. 1984. "The Efficacy and Cost-Effectiveness of Vehicle Inspection." *Journal of Transport Economics and Policy* 18, no. 2:145.

MACKAY, M. 1985. "Two Years' Experience with the Seat Belt Law in Britain." SAE Technical Papers, series no. 851234, 15 pages.

MAIN, T. 1985. "An Economic Evaluation of Child Restraints." *Journal of Transport Economics and Policy* 19:23.

MULLER, A. 1980. "Evaluations of the Cost and Benefit of Motorcycle Helmet Laws." *American Journal of Public Health* 70:586–92.

———. 1984. "Daytime Headlight Operation and Motorcyclist Fatalities." *Accident Analysis and Prevention* 16:1–18.

MULLER, A., and T. J. REUTZEL. 1984. "Willingness to Pay for Reduction in Fatality Risk: An Exploratory Survey." *American Journal of Public Health* 74:808–11.

NAS. 1984. *55: A Decade of Experience*. Transportation Research Board, Washington, D.C: National Academy of Sciences.

NASS. 1981. *Report on Traffic Accidents and Injuries for 1979–1980*. Washington, D.C: U.S. Department of Transportation, NHTSA.

NEWMAN, R. J., and I. S. JONES. 1984. "A Prospective Study of 413 Consecutive Car Occupants with Chest Injuries." *Journal of Trauma* 24:129–35.

NEWMAN, R. J., and S. RASTOGI. 1984. "Rupture of the Thoracic Aorta and Its Relationship to Road Traffic Accident Characteristics." *Injury* 15:296–99.

NHTSA. 1981. *Highway Safety Needs Study: 1981 Update of 1976 Report to Congress*. DOT-HS-806-283. Washington, D.C: U.S. Department of Transportation.

NHTSA. 1983. *The Economic Cost to Society of Traffic Accidents*. Washington, D.C: U. S. Department of Transportation.

NORDHAUS, W. 1981. "Comments on Proposed Rulemaking, FMVSS 208: Occupant Crash Protection." NHTSA Docket 74–14, Notice 22, Washington, D.C.

NORSTROM, T. 1983. "Law Enforcement and Alcohol Consumption Policy as Countermeasures Against Drunken Driving: Possibilities and Limitations." *Accident Analysis and Prevention* 15:513–21.

NSC. 1984. *Accident Facts*, Chicago Ill.: National Safety Council.

PELTZMAN, S. 1975. "The Effects of Automobile Safety Regulation." *Journal of Political Economy* 83:677–725.

PREUSSER, D. F., W. A. LEAF, K. B. DEBARTOLO, R. D. BLOMBERG, and M. M. LEVY. 1982. "The Effect of Right-Turn-on-Red on Pedestrian and Bicyclist Accidents." *Journal of Safety Research* 13, no. 2:45.

PREUSSER, D. F., A. F. WILLIAMS, P. L. ZADOR, and R. D. BLOMBERG. 1984. "The Effect of Curfew Laws on Motor Vehicle Crashes." *Law and Policy* 6, no. 1:115–28.

PREUSSER, D. F., A. F. WILLIAMS, AND A. K. LUND. 1985. "Driver Licensing Age and Lifestyles of 16 Year Olds." *American Journal of Public Health* 75:358.

RICCI, L. 1979. *National Crash Severity Study Statistics*. DOT-HS-805-227. Washington D.C.: Department of Transportation, NHTSA.

ROBERTSON, L. S. 1980. "Crash Involvement of Teenage Drivers When Drivers Education Is Eliminated from High School." *American Journal of Public Health* 70:599.

ROSS, H. L., H. KLETTE, and R. MCCLEARY. 1984. "Liberalization and Rationalization of Drunk-Driving Laws in Scandinavia." *Accident Analysis and Prevention* 16:471–87.

ROSS, H. L., R. MCCLEARY, and T. EPPERLEIN. 1981–82. "Deterrence of Drinking and Driving in France: An Evaluation of the Law of July 12, 1978." *Law and Society Review* 16, no. 3:345.

ROWE, W. 1983. "Design and Performance Standards." *Medical Devices: Measurements, Quality Assurance, and Standards*, C. A. Caceres et al. (eds.). Philadelphia: ASTM, pp. 29–40.

SALZBERG, P. M., and S. P. PAULSRUDE. 1984. "An Evaluation of Washington's Driving While Intoxicated Law: Effect on Drunk Driving Recidivism." *Journal of Safety Research* 15, no. 3:117.

SMART, C. N., and C. R. SANDERS. 1976. *The Costs of Motor Vehicle and Related Spinal Cord Injuries*. Washington D.C.: Insurance Institute for Highway Safety.

SOLOMON, K. A., P. E. PERKINS, and S. RESETAR. 1985. *Improving Automotive Safety: The Role of Industry, the Government, and the Driver*. Rand Corporation, P-7069, 27 pages.

THOMPSON, F. 1985. "Regulating Motor Vehicle Safety Maintenance: Can We Make It Cost-Effective?" *Journal of Health Politics, Policy and Law* 9, no. 4:695.

TOFANY, V. L. 1981. "Life Is Best at 55." *Traffic Quarterly* 35, no. 1:5.

VAN MATRE, J. G., G. A. OVERSTREET JR. 1982. "Motor Vehicle Inspection and Accident Mortality: A Reexamination." *Journal of Risk and Insurance* 49, no. 2:423.

VOTEY, H. L., JR., 1984. "Recent Evidence from Scandinavia on Deterring Alcohol Impaired Driving." *Accident Analysis and Prevention* 16:123-28.

VOTEY, H. L., JR., and P. SHAPIRO, 1983. "Highway Accidents in Sweden: Modelling the Process of Drunken Driving Behavior and Control." *Accident Analysis and Prevention* 15:523–33.

WAGENAAR, A. C. 1982. "Preventing Highway Crashes by Raising the Legal Minimum Age for Drinking: An Empirical Confirmation." *Journal of Safety Research* 13, no. 2:57.

———. 1985. "Mandatory Child Restraint Laws: Impact on Childhood Injuries Due to Traffic Crashes." *Journal of Safety Research* 16, no. 1:9.

WALSH, P. V., G. A. TROTTER. 1979–80. "Fracture of the Thyroid Cartilage Associated with Full Face Integral Crash Helmet." *Injury* 2:47–8.

WILLIAMS, A. F., P. L. ZADOR, S. S. HARRIS, and R. S. KARPF. 1983. "The Effect of Raising the Minimum Drinking Age on Involvement in Fatal Crashes." *Journal of Legal Studies* 12:169–80.

WINSTON, C. and F. MANNERING. 1984. "Consumer Demand for Automobile Safety." *American Economic Review* 74:316–19.

ZADOR, P., J. MOSHMAN, and L. MARCUS. 1982. "Adoption of Right Turn on Red: Effects on Crashes at Signalized Intersections." *Accident Analysis and Prevention* 14:219–34.

Chapter 2

INJURY REDUCTION AND BELT USE ASSOCIATED WITH OCCUPANT RESTRAINT LAWS

by B. J. Campbell and Frances A. Campbell

Introduction

The United States may legitimately claim to be a world leader in the prevention of motor vehicle injuries, but in the adoption of seat belt use laws, we are far behind other industrialized nations. As long ago as 1970, parliamentarians in Victoria, Australia, enacted the world's first seat belt law. In contrast, New York became the first American state to adopt such a law in late 1984, by which time the list of other nations with belt laws was long indeed (see Table 2–1).

One reason for the delay in passing seat belt legislation in the United States may have been a lack of early advocacy on the part of traffic safety leadership groups. In the absence of vigorous support by leadership groups, there was little movement toward seat belt laws during the 1960s and 70s. Illustrative is the fact that,

---

Some of the analysis in this chapter is treated in more detail in B. J. Campbell, J. R. Stewart, and Frances A. Campbell, "1985–1986 Experience with Belt Laws in the United States" (Chapel Hill, N.C.: Highway Safety Research Center, University of North Carolina at Chapel Hill, 1987); and B. J. Campbell and Frances A. Campbell, *Seat Belt Law Experience in Four Foreign Countries Compared to the United States* (Falls Church, Va.: AAA Foundation for Traffic Safety, 1986).

Table 2–1 Countries with Laws Requiring Seat Belt Use

Country	Date Instituted	Usage Rates (%)
Australia	1/1/70	87
Austria	7/15/76	33
Belgium	6/1/75	87
Brazil	1977	
Bulgaria	7/1/76	
Canada (7 prov)	75–84	50–60
Czechoslovakia	7/75	66
Denmark	1/1/76	75
Finland	7/1/75	93
France	7/1/83	78
Greece	12/16/79	
Hungary	7/1/77	
Iceland	1983	60
Ireland	2/1/79	46
Israel	7/1/75	70
Ivory Coast	1970	
Japan	12/1/71	21
Luxembourg	6/1/71	
Malawi	1982	
Malaysia	4/1/79	
Netherlands	6/1/75	67
New Zealand	6/1/72	67
Norway	9/1/75	90
Puerto Rico	1/74	
Portugal	1982	
South Africa	12/1/77	62
Spain	10/3/74	67
Sweden	1/1/75	80
Switzerland	1/1/76	81
Turkey	1982	
United Kingdom	1/83	95
USSR	1/1/76	
West Germany	1/1/76	54
Yugoslavia	1/1/77	

Source: Grimm (1984).

in the late 1960s, the newly created National Highway Safety Bureau (NHSB) of the United States Department of Transportation (DOT) promulgated 17 different state standards touching almost every area of highway safety, none of which had anything to do with seat belt use. It was not until 1984 that, for the first time, DOT publicly endorsed seat belt laws.

Leadership groups in the private sector also largely ignored such laws until recently. The American Public Health Association endorsed belt laws only in the fall of 1983, and the Consumer's Union, in November 1984. The American Automobile Association and the American Medical Association made such endorsements in 1985. The auto industry only recently supported the passage of such laws. General Motors, for example, endorsed seat belt mandates in late 1983 (Campbell and Campbell, 1986).

One factor that almost certainly delayed consideration of such laws was the division of opinion over the desirability of automatic restraint systems such as air bags, as opposed to mandated use of seat belts. This argument, which appears not to have been a significant factor in foreign countries, was a divisive factor in the United States for years. It seemed to create a stalemate that helped to block implementation of either approach.

If the air bag issue delayed the passage of belt laws, the success of child safety seat laws almost certainly helped to create a climate of public acceptance for them. The first such child protection law took effect in Tennessee in 1978, and in 1985 Wyoming became the 50th state to follow suit. There was relatively little opposition to the enactment of this protective legislation for young children.

By 1984, with growing support from the federal government, other key national organizations, and the auto industry, adult belt laws began to be passed in the United States. As of late 1987, the country has undergone a remarkable change in public policy regarding safety belts. About three-fourths of the population is now covered by adult belt use laws. Moreover, with automatic restraint systems also now a reality, the era of occupant restraint seems upon us. Table 2–2 shows the current status of belt laws.

Fatality Changes Associated with Belt Laws

A number of analysts have examined the relationship between belt laws and casualty reduction in the United States, as was done earlier in several foreign countries (see reviews in Campbell, Stewart, and Campbell, 1987; Wagenaar, Maybee, and Sullivan, in press; Campbell and Campbell, 1986; and Hedlund, 1986). One such analysis, which examines trends in national fatalities in the years 1975 through 1986, is presented in this section. The data are from the Fatal Accident Reporting System (FARS) maintained by the National Highway Traffic Safety Administration (NHTSA). This analysis compares fatalities within a group covered by seat belt laws (front seat occupants of cars, light trucks, and vans) with those in another group (the remainder of those in the FARS file). Fatality trends for these two groups (called the Covered group and the

Table 2–2   Years in Which Seat Belt Use Laws Became Effective

1984	1985	1986	1987	1988
New York	New Jersey	Connecticut	Oklahoma	Virginia
	Michigan	New Mexico	Indiana	
	Illinois	California	Montana	
	Texas	Massachusetts (repealed)	Colorado	
	Nebraska (repealed)	Tennessee	Nevada	
	Missouri	Utah	Oregon	
	North Carolina	Ohio		
	District of Columbia	Louisiana		
	Hawaii	Iowa		
		Maryland		
		Washington		
		Idaho		
		Kansas		
		Florida		
		Minnesota		

Other group) were examined before and after belt laws took effect. Fatality trends in these same groups within nonlaw states were used as a control by expressing the experience in the law states as a proportion of that of nonlaw states, month by month. Time series analyses (Box and Jenkins, 1976) for Covered and Other groups were performed on these proportions.

Our assumption was that any change in fatality trends at the onset of a belt law would be in the form of an abrupt, one-time shift, such as defined by o-x-y-b in the schematic shown in Figure 2–1. It is assumed that the benefit would be described by the area x-y-b-a-x if the effect persists, or x-y-a-x if the effect fades. One

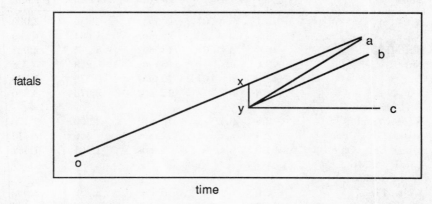

Figure 2-1   Schematic Representation of Possible Casualty Trends Pre-
and Post-Law.

would not expect a change in slope like o-x-y-c, because that would imply a progressively more effective impact of belt laws over time.

FARS data available through 1986 allowed analysis of pre- and postlaw experience in 24 states plus the District of Columbia. For purposes of this analysis, states were grouped according to the effective date of their law. Eleven such groupings were defined and examined separately. Some groups consist of single states; others contain two or more states. The results are given in Table 2–3. Overall, observed fatalities among Covered occupants in the 25 belt law jurisdictions were 6.6 percent less than the number forecast for these states. This 6.6 percent improvement amounts to an estimated savings of 1,300 lives in the time period in question.

In five of the eleven groups tested, statistically significant intervention effects were found—that is, there was a significant change in the trend at the time the law took effect. This change occurred in January 1985 in New York, in March 1985 in New Jersey, in July 1985 in Michigan-Illinois, and in September 1985 in Texas. Thus, in all these states the significant trend break corresponded to the month of the law's onset. In five other groups of states, there was an improvement in fatalities relative to the number forecast, but in these five the intervention effect did not attain statistical significance.

Nine of the 11 groups showed net reductions in fatality levels below that forecast on the basis of past trends. Texas had the largest

Table 2–3   Time Series Results for Fatalities Among Covered Occupants

States	Percent Change	Interv. Signif.	Period of Forecast	Fatalities Forecast	Actual Fatalities
N.Y.	−10.1	$p < .01$	24 mos.	2,336	2,099
N.J.	−8.7	$p = .01$	22 mos.	1,094	999
Ill., Mich.	−6.0	$p < .01$	18 mos.	3,113	2,927
Nebr.	+3.6	n.s.	16 mos.	249	258
Tex.	−18.6	$p < .01$	16 mos.	3,378	2,749
Mo., N.C.	+8.8	n.s.	15 mos.	2,078	2,260
D.C., Hawaii, Conn., N. Mex., Calif.	−3.8	n.s.	12 mos.	3,300	3,175
Mass.	−9.4	n.s.	12 mos.	456	413
Tenn., Utah, Ohio, La., Iowa, Md., Wash., Idaho, Kans., Fla.	−1.0	n.s.	8 mos.	1,465	1,451
	−6.0	n.s.	6 mos.	2,130	2,002
Minn.	−17.2	$p = .10$	5 mos.	198	164
Total	−6.6			19,797	18,497

favorable change, showing an 18.6 percent reduction. New York fatalities were about 10 percent below forecast. In New Jersey, the improvement was 8.7 percent; in Illinois-Michigan, fatalities were 6.0 percent less than forecast.

In two groups, observed fatalities exceeded the number forecast by the time series model. Nebraska fatalities exceeded the amount forecast only slightly, but in the group consisting of Missouri–North Carolina, fatalities exceeded the forecast to a considerable degree (8.8 percent above forecast—almost 200 fatalities the wrong way).

The contemporaneous fatality trends in the Other group (not covered by the law) provide data against which to compare those in the Covered group within seat belt law states. Accordingly, time series analyses were performed on fatality trends in the Other group within those states where there was a statistically significant intervention effect for the Covered group. Table 2–4 presents results for New York, New Jersey, Michigan-Illinois combined, and Texas, and reveals that, within the Other group in these states, there was no concurrent favorable change in fatality and no significant break in the trend associated with the law's onset date. In these five states, Other fatalities were 2.0 percent above the numbers forecast, whereas in the Covered groups of these same states, deaths were 11.6 percent below forecast.

To summarize, analysis of the FARS data reveals that, among Covered occupants in 24 belt law jurisdictions, fatalities were 6.6 percent lower than the number forecast from past trends. Among Other victims, observed fatalities were 2 percent above the forecast level. Further, in several belt law states there was a break in the trend for Covered occupants significantly associated with the month of the law's onset, but no such significant shifts in fatality trends were seen among the Other group.

Injury Reduction Associated with Belt Laws

It may be that belt laws will produce a greater societal benefit in terms of injury reduction than fatality reduction. Injuries are much

Table 2–4　Time Series Results for Fatalities Among the Other Group

States	Percent Change	Interv. Signif.	Period of Forecast	Fatalities Forecast	Actual Fatalities
N.Y.	+2.8	n.s.	24 mos.	1,879	1,932
N.J.	+6.9	n.s.	22 mos.	782	836
Ill., Mich.	+2.7	n.s.	18 mos.	1,808	1,857
Tex.	−1.6	n.s.	16 mos.	1,827	1,797
Total	+2.0			6,296	6,422

more numerous than fatalities, and the worst of them constitute a considerable public burden. It is not possible to carry out the same sort of national analysis of injury reduction as was possible for fatality reduction because there is no comparable national data base. However, the authors have either analyzed or obtained analyses by others of the statewide injury data from five belt law states: Illinois, Michigan, North Carolina, New York, and Texas. Results for each state are presented below.

Illinois

Data were provided by the Illinois Department of Transportation, covering monthly injury frequencies for five years before the July 1, 1985, onset of the Illinois law, and for 18 months since that time. From this data set it was possible to determine the number of serious plus fatal injuries sustained by motor vehicle occupants in that state before and after the onset of the seat belt law. A time series analysis using these injury frequencies revealed a highly significant intervention effect associated with the month the Illinois law took effect. This implies that the law had a positive effect upon injuries, even though the injury data could not be confined solely to front seat occupants, the group specifically covered by the law.

By projecting the injuries forecast had there been no intervention and contrasting that projection with the observed number, it was possible to estimate a 6.2 percent decrease in serious injuries over the 18-month postlaw period. This amounts to about 1,861 such injuries saved per year in Illinois. This injury savings projects to approximately 39,000 saved per year nationally if all states had the same experience as Illinois. Figure 2–2 is a graph of monthly serious plus fatal injuries in Illinois during the time period in question.

Michigan

Wagenaar, Maybee, and Sullivan (1987) reported a significant change in Michigan crash injuries associated with the effective date of their seat belt law. Using the frequency of any injury to any occupant as the factor tested, they performed a time series analysis on the first six months of the Michigan law (July–December 1985), contrasted with monthly prelaw data beginning January 1978. These authors reported a reduction in injuries of 12.1 percent, an estimated savings of 7,278 injuries. If one projects Michigan's half-

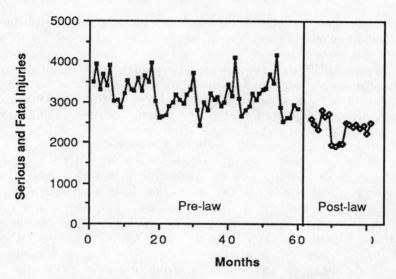

Figure 2-2   Illinois Serious Injuries, Pre- and Post-Law.

year experience to the entire nation, there would be an estimated national savings of over one-third million injuries annually.

North Carolina

Monthly statewide crash data from North Carolina were used for this analysis, beginning with January 1981. As in the foregoing analyses of fatal crash data, a Covered group was defined in which the trend in injuries was contrasted to that in three Other groups not subject to the law. These three Other groups were (1) rear seat occupants of covered vehicles, (2) occupants of vehicles not covered by the law, and (3) all other persons in crashes (mainly nonoccupants such as pedestrians and cyclists).

The analyses separately addressed the two phases of the North Carolina law. During Phase 1, enforcement was limited to the use of warning tickets. The warning phase lasted fifteen months, and was characterized by belt use of 42 to 44 percent. Phase 2 saw full enforcement of the law, with a maximum fine of $25 for noncompliance. Six months of Phase 2 casualty data are currently available—a period when belt use was 64 to 78 percent.

Phase 1 was marked by a modest favorable shift in injury trends. An improvement of 6.9 percent in serious and greater injuries was seen. When the injury range is extended to include moderate or worse injuries, an improvement of 3.2 percent is seen. Intervention tests performed for the month of the law's onset showed marginal significance ($p < .10$ one-tailed test). For the Other groups, the changes were of lesser magnitude, and no intervention effects were seen.

The onset of Phase 2 in January of 1987 was marked by an abrupt and pronounced further improvement in injury among Covered occupants. For moderate and greater injuries, the improvement was 9.8 percent below forecast. For serious and greater injuries, the improvement was 13.6 percent below forecast. The intervention effect was highly significant in both instances.

This improvement in injury incidence in the Covered group contrasts to the trends seen in two of the three Other groups in North Carolina. For Nonoccupants and for Rear-seat occupants of covered cars, there was a modest decrease in injuries, but the decrease was not significantly associated with the January onset of the law. Of greater interest is the behavior of the third Other subgroup, consisting of occupants of noncovered vehicles (older cars and certain trucks). In this group moderate and greater injuries were 11.8 percent below forecast, and the January intervention effect was significant. With regard to serious and greater injuries, the improvement was 6.8 percent below forecast, but the intervention test was not statistically significant.

Though the law did not cover occupants riding in these classes of vehicles, it may be that onset of full enforcement of the law nevertheless changed their belt use. Given that belt use in the population at risk reached 78 percent, it would not necessarily be surprising to see an increase in the number of buckled occupants, even in vehicles not covered by the law. There are as yet, however, no data to verify this idea. In any event, the change in this group is not counted in the estimate of belt law benefit for North Carolina.

The North Carolina injury changes affected a large number of people. During Phase 2 the benefit is estimated at about 1,978 serious injuries prevented in a year, which projects to a savings of about 75,000 per year nationally. With respect to moderate and greater injuries, the North Carolina savings is estimated at 3,754 in a year, an amount that projects to 140,000 per year nationally. Figure 2–3 depicts Covered occupants and shows the percent serious and greater injury during the prelaw, Phase 1, and Phase 2 periods.

New York

The Highway Safety Research Center (HSRC) analyzed statewide injury data from New York for the years 1984–1986. Because of the

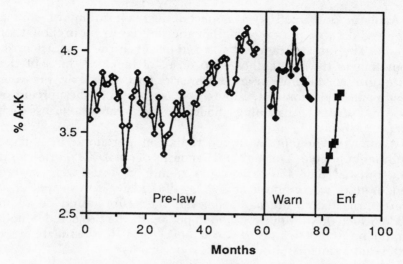

Figure 2-3 North Carolina Serious Injuries, Pre- and Post-Law.

limited prelaw data available, the postlaw forecast of injury was based only on the single year prior to onset of the law. The data available also made it necessary to confine the analysis to drivers only.

Among Covered drivers, the trend for moderate or greater injury and for serious or greater injury improved significantly at the onset of the law—that is, such injuries occurred at levels substantially below the levels forecast had there been no law. In contrast, injuries among the Other drivers either stayed the same as forecast, or rose.

Again, this benefit was realized by large numbers of people. If one projects the New York driver experience nationwide, the estimate is that about 40,000 drivers annually would be spared moderate or greater injuries as a result of a seat belt law. If the estimate is extended to all front seat occupants, the savings might be as great as 50,000 per year.

Texas

Statewide Texas crash data included 56 months of prelaw data beginning with January 1981, and 16 months of postlaw data beginning in September 1985. The Covered group consisted of drivers of vehicles covered under the Texas belt law. The Other group was drivers of vehicles not covered by the law, plus operators of motorcycles or mopeds, bicyclists, and pedestrians.

Analysis confirmed a pronounced decrease in injury among Covered drivers, but no such dramatic shift occurred in the Other group. The intervention test was significant in the former (corresponding to the September 1985 onset of the law), but not the latter group. Moderate or greater injuries for Covered drivers were 9 percent below forecast. Figure 2–4 is a graph of the percent of Covered drivers sustaining moderate or greater injuries each month in Texas.

Again, the benefit in injury reduction pertained to a large number of people. During the 16 months of postlaw experience, it is estimated that 456 drivers per month in Texas were spared moderate or worse injuries by virtue of the law. If this experience were projected to the national level, the result would be about 80,000 such driver injuries avoided per year. The projected benefit would be 100,000 injuries saved per year if the estimate were extended to include other front seat occupants.

*   *   *

In summary, injury data from these five states indicate substantial downward shifts among Covered occupants of motor vehicles with the onset of seat belt laws. In the three states for which Other groups were available for comparison, similar downward shifts were generally not seen. In the one instance, there was a significant downward shift among occupants of vehicle classes excluded from the North Carolina law. However, in view of the high belt

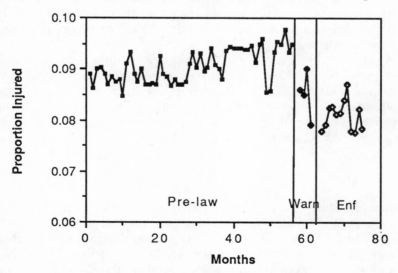

Figure 2-4 Texas Moderate Injuries, Pre- and Post-Law.

use prevailing in North Carolina, it may be reasonable to suppose that belt use increased in these vehicles too, but there is no direct evidence on the matter. Table 2–5 gives injury reduction figures by state.

If the injury ranges considered here are ordered from broadest (any injury at all) to narrowest (serious to fatal), it becomes apparent that the estimates are reasonably consistent in that smaller absolute savings are projected for progressively more severe injury categories, as is shown below:

- Projected from *any* injury in Michigan, about 330,000 slight to fatal injuries might be saved each year nationally.
- Projected from Moderate or greater injuries in Texas, New York, and North Carolina, 40,000 to 140,000 such injuries might be saved each year nationally.
- Projected from Serious or greater injuries in Illinois and North Carolina, 39,000 to 75,000 such injuries might be saved each year nationally.

Changes in Belt Use Associated with the Law

In virtually every state, a substantial increase in belt use followed the effective date of the law, doubling or even tripling prelaw usage in most cases. In general, statewide belt use figures in each state are determined by direct observation. Survey personnel are stationed at numerous representative sites around the state to observe belt use in passing vehicles. In the 25 belt law jurisdictions for which data are available ("latest use" column in Table 2–6), the population weighted belt use is 48 percent overall. Among these states, six report usage rates of 60 percent or above, but seven report levels below 40 percent (not including Massachusetts and Nebraska where the laws have been repealed).

Some of the state-by-state variation seen here may be a function of differing survey procedures. Not all states use the same observing and sampling methods, and some of the available "overall" figures are not based on representative samples. The Texas data,

Table 2–5 Injury Reduction Percentages by State

Illinois	− 6.2	serious injury reduction	intervention significant
Michigan	− 12.1	any injury reduction	intervention significant
North Carolina	− 13.6	serious injury reduction	intervention significant
New York	− 6.2	moderate injury reduction	intervention significant
Texas	− 9.0	moderate injury reduction	intervention significant

Table 2–6   Belt Use Survey Results by State

State	Pre-law Baseline Belt Use (%)	Highest Belt Use (%)	Latest Belt Use (%)
California	18	47	47
Connecticut	25	56	56
Colorado	18		
D.C.		55	55
Florida	22	60	60
Hawaii	33	73	64
Idaho	16	27	27
Illinois	16	47	47
Indiana	20	52	52
Iowa	18	63	63
Kansas	10	44	44
Louisiana	12	35	35
Maryland	30	74	66
Massachusetts	20	37	25 (repeal)
Michigan	20	58	47
Minnesota	20	33	32
Missouri	10	34	40
Montana	33		
Nebraska	11	45	29 (repeal)
Nevada	21		
New Jersey	18	42	41
New Mexico	12	53	50
New York	16	57	48
North Carolina	25	77	64
Ohio	16	48	41
Oklahoma	16	41	35
Oregon	35		
Tennessee		28	28
Texas	15	66	60
Utah	18	22	22
Virginia	32		
Washington		36	51
Latest average, population weighted (less Ma and Nb)			48%

for example, are confined to city observations, and the Maryland data are not portrayed by Maryland officials as representative of the entire state. Some figures are based on observations of drivers only, while others are based on all front seat occupants. In every case, however, the surveys are based on large numbers of observations taken at a considerable number of sites, and they constitute the best currently available indication of belt use in the respective states.

The Association Between Enforcement and Belt Usage

It seems logical that there would be an association between the level of enforcement of belt laws and level of belt usage in compliance. This section examines that association within two groups of states which differ in enforcement practice: (1) eight states with *primary enforcement* policies in which the officer may stop a motorist solely on the basis of a seat belt law violation; (2) twelve states with *secondary enforcement* policies under which a seat belt law violation may be addressed only if the officer has stopped the motorist for some other purpose.

Enforcement data were collected by means of a mail survey sent to the highway patrol or state police (Campbell, 1987). The data are confined to statistics on citations and do not reflect final adjudication. The data are drawn from state police agencies only, because local enforcement data are rarely assembled on a statewide basis. Belt use data were assembled from the Governor's Highway Safety Representative in belt law states, the office that customarily coordinates these surveys.

From information on belt usage and enforcement level, the statistical association between the two was determined. For purposes of this analysis, belt usage values most concurrent with the time period covered by available citation figures were used. Thus, the latest usage figures were not used in every case.

Results

To examine the strength of association between enforcement levels and usage levels, the plots for primary and secondary enforcement states are depicted in Figures 2–5 and 2–6. Although these regressions are based on relatively few plotting points, the individual plotting points represent thousands of observations in both dimensions. Note that for primary enforcement states, the association is stronger than for secondary enforcement states, with a tau of + .86 for the former versus + .43 for the latter, although both tau values are significantly different from zero. The regression slope of the primary states is somewhat steeper than that of the secondary states—.029 versus .024, and the intercept values are different—45 versus 32 percent.

The analysis thus suggests two additive factors at work: first, in both primary and secondary enforcement states, belt usage is higher in the presence of higher levels of enforcement; second, for a given level of enforcement, usage is higher in primary than in secondary enforcement states.

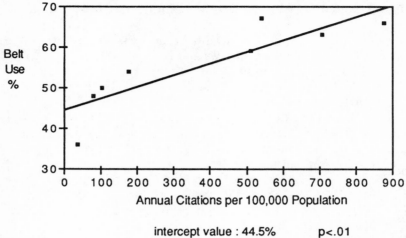

intercept value : 44.5%   p<.01
slope   : .029
Kendall's Tau   : + .86   p<.01

Figure 2-5 Belt Usage versus Enforcement for Eight Primary Enforcement
States.

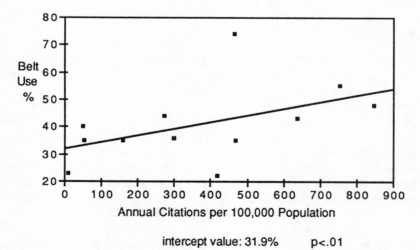

intercept value: 31.9%   p<.01
slope   : .024
Kendall's Tau : + .43   p<.03

Figure 2-6 Belt Usage versus Enforcement in Twelve Secondary Enforcement
States.

Does Increased Enforcement Produce Higher Belt Use?

The above analysis merely describes the statistical association between enforcement and usage; however, other evidence bears on the causal relationship. There is a logical basis for assuming that enforcement of a belt law directly influences compliance. Moreover, in a number of instances, changes in enforcement (upward or down) have been followed by immediate changes in belt usage. The following examples are illustrative.

In Elmira, New York, where a highly publicized special enforcement effort was undertaken, belt use increased from 49 to 77 percent immediately during and following the campaign, and had declined only to 66 percent a few months later (Williams et al., 1986). In Nebraska and Massachusetts, after repeal of the law, belt use fell to levels lower than is seen in virtually any active belt law state—29 and 25 percent, respectively. When the governor of Illinois recently announced a change in the de facto secondary enforcement policy, a partial survey in that state indicated a concurrent rise in use rates.

Thus, as common sense would suggest, there is evidence to indicate that enforcement affects compliance. That does not mean there is a one-to-one relationship between changes in enforcement and changes in belt usage; clearly, the matter is not so simple. For example, if belt use were sufficiently high as to make it difficult for officers to spot violators, then such a relationship could not be documented. However, with average belt use less than 50 percent, locating candidates for enforcement action is not difficult. There does, however, appear to be evidence to support the notion that if the public believes there will be *no* consequences of ignoring the belt law, compliance is apt to be lower.

It is also of interest to consider the changes in use rates seen when enforcement begins immediately after the law takes effect in contrast to the situation when there is a significant warning period before full enforcement. In Michigan, full enforcement began immediately with the formal onset of the law. Prelaw surveys revealed percent usage in the low to mid-20s, with a sharp increase to near 60 percent immediately after onset of the law. Thereafter, percent belt use fell to the mid-40s and has remained relatively constant since (see Figure 2–7).

Other states had formal or informal "grace" periods before full enforcement was instituted. The experience in Kansas illustrates one pattern of results seen in this case: belt usage, low to begin with, doubled from the prelaw to postlaw period, then increased again approximately a year later when full enforcement began (see Figure 2–8).

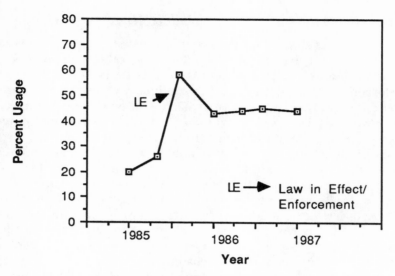

Figure 2-7   Michigan Belt Use.

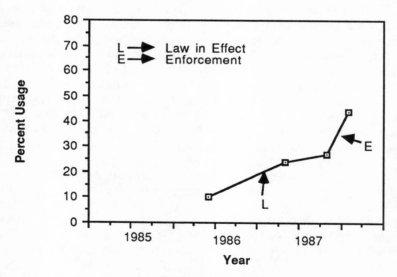

Figure 2-8   Kansas Belt Use.

North Carolina shows still another pattern, depicted in Figure
2–9. There was an appreciable increase over baseline use at onset
of the law, and the higher level was rather steady during the 15
months when written warning tickets were given out at a rather
intense rate. As in Kansas, after full enforcement began, there was
a second, sharper, rise. Following the second increase, however,

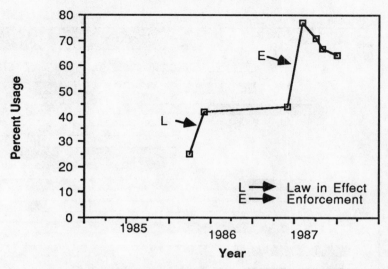

Figure 2-9   North Carolina Belt Use.

there has been a decline, despite the fact that the level of enforcement appears to be steady. It should be noted that North Carolina's
rate is nevertheless high relative to overall national experience.

The apparent link between enforcement and belt usage suggests
the possibility that the full effectiveness of belt laws has not yet
been realized. Many states did not yet pursue full enforcement
during 1986, the latest time for which national fatality data are
available. Figure 2–10, a chart showing when full enforcement
began in belt law states, shows that only in 1987 does full enforcement prevail in most of the states.

Factors That Produce Large Shifts in National Fatalities

Prior to the actual passage of seat belt laws, various advocates
made predictions that large downward shifts in the national fatality
toll would be produced by adoption of such laws. For example, it
has been said that if seat belts, or air bags, or a combination of
both were universally available and used, that 10,000 lives might
be saved per year. Presumably, supporters of seat belt laws are
hopefully waiting for that to happen, and opponents are gleefully
waiting for it not to happen.

It would perhaps be useful here to consider the periods in U.S.
traffic safety history when major, rapid shifts in fatality trends did
occur. As shown in Table 2–7, only three times over the years have

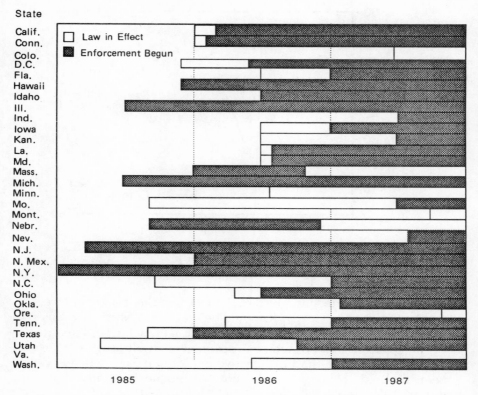

Figure 2-10   Belt Use Law Onset and Enforcement.

fatalities increased by 5,000 or more deaths in a relatively short time and, conversely, only four times have deaths fallen by 7,000 or more in a short time (National Safety Council, 1986).

It is only possible, of course, to speculate on the reasons for these massive changes. By the 1930s, automobile accidents were

Table 2–7   Temporal Trends in Motor Vehicle Deaths

Period	Years	Direction	Number of Deaths
1937–1938	1	down	7,000
1940–1941	1	up	5,000
1941–1942	1	down	16,000
1944–1946	2	up	9,000
1961–1966	5	up	15,000
1973–1975	2	down	9,000
1981–1983	2	down	9,000

Source: Accident Facts (1986).

already a considerable problem in the United States, and by 1937 annual deaths reached 39,643. The death rate per hundred million driving miles was more than five times greater than today (14.68 vs. 2.58). There was a large decrease (down 7,000) in 1937–38, seemingly not related to changes in exposure, for the mileage exposure before and after the decrease stayed virtually the same. The depths of the Great Depression coincided with this period. The upswing in deaths just before World War II may have reflected the economic expansion on the eve of the war and the consequent increase in exposure. There was an increase of 10 percent in mileage during the same period, but fatalities went up even more (up 5,000).

The largest downswing in our nation's history (a decrease of 16,000 lives over a single-year period) happened early in World War II, when mileage exposure dropped by more than one-third. Gas rationing, tire rationing, a 35 MPH speed limit, and millions of young men in the armed services and off the highways all coincided with this period; all these factors presumably contributed. Actually, fatalities per unit exposure were about the same as earlier; thus this improvement appears to have been almost entirely exposure-driven. After the war, at the time of demobilization, there was an increase of 9,000 traffic fatalities within two years. The reduced mileage exposure seen during the war was reversed. As with the previous large decline, the increase in fatalities was largely exposure-driven, but fatalities actually increased somewhat less than exposure would have indicated, suggesting the simultaneous influence of other factors.

The next upswing in fatalities was very large, though spread over a longer period; there was an increase of nearly 15,000 in fatalities from 1961 to 1966. In 1961, the actual number of deaths in the United States was 38,091—fewer than the 39,643 recorded 24 years earlier in 1937. Thus, despite the growth in population and cars from the 1930s to 1961, the death *rate* per hundred million miles had fallen so much that the raw number of fatalities remained relatively constant. Within the next five years, however, the toll soared such that in 1966 the raw number of deaths was 53,041.

This rise is described by two phenomena: first, a great increase in cars and mileage exposure, and second, by a plateau in the improvement in mileage death rate. For approximately nine years the mileage death rate did not fall. In 1961, the death rate per hundred million vehicle miles was 5.16. In 1969, it was 5.21. This long-term stagnation in the death rate was unique to that point in history—a time when car ownership was soaring, speed limits were high, and powerful cars were a central fact of car marketing and owner preference. It was probably no coincidence that, during the same period, calls for an increased federal role in highway safety were growing more urgent, finally culminating in the creation of the National Highway Safety Bureau in 1967.

The downswing in fatalities in 1973–1975 reflected a combination of the oil embargo, the related severe recession, and the 55 MPH speed limit enacted in response. In that time, annual deaths dropped by about 9,000, despite the fact that exposure did not decrease proportionately. Likewise, during the recession of 1981–1983, a drop in fatalities of 9,000 occurred, though exposure remained much the same.

The point is that the occasional very large changes in U.S. highway fatalities have been "powered" by major societal forces— wars, recessions, or periods of great economic growth. It has not yet been possible to produce fatality changes of comparable magnitude by imposition of any specific highway safety countermeasure. Viewed from this perspective, it seems unlikely that seat belt laws, as powerful a measure as they constitute, can be expected to effect dramatic, large downward shifts in fatalities comparable to those associated with such major historical events.

Why Aren't Belt Law Benefits Greater?

From the analyses presented earlier in this chapter, it appears that at present, belt laws in the United States have produced a fatality improvement of about 7 percent, with a slightly greater improvement in injury—approximately 10 percent. Those who deal in countermeasure evaluation recognize that a 10 percent reduction represents a good response to a single countermeasure. Nevertheless, research suggests that, with universal use, casualties might be reduced by as much as 40 percent. Since to date, only a 7 percent reduction has been realized, it is useful to attempt to account for this difference between projected and actual benefits. The North Carolina situation may be used to illustrate several factors possibly related to the lower benefit rates:

1. Belt laws do not apply to all persons at risk for injury or death on the highways. The North Carolina belt law exempts rear seat occupants; it exempts all commercial and farm vehicles being used in commerce; it exempts older cars; it provides for medical exemptions; it exempts slow-moving delivery vehicles. In addition, the law does not apply to bicycle, pedestrian, or motorcycle crashes. All in all, 30 percent or more of those in crashes fall into categories not covered by the North Carolina seat belt law.

2. Not everyone covered by the law uses the belt. In North Carolina surveys during the summer of 1987, belt use among persons covered by the law was 64 percent. Obviously, the potential benefit is again reduced, in that a maximum of 64 percent of the above 70 percent of victims were buckled up. Further, the 64 percent represents a growth from a prelaw baseline of as much as 25 percent. Benefits from the prelaw belt use are hidden away in the prelaw casualty trends. Thus, there was a net growth in belt use of only about half the population at risk (less actually). Half of the above 70 percent is 35 percent.

3. Belt effectiveness in reducing injury and death is about 40 to 50 percent; 40 to 50 percent of the above 35 percent is about 14 to 17 percent.

4. State population and driving mileage is growing. If miles driven increase about 5 percent each year, then, other things being equal, fatalities would similarly increase. That growth would offset some of the belt law benefits.

5. As noted in the previous section, changes in the economy exercise a heavy influence on road deaths—beyond that accounted for by changes in driving mileage. During the recession of the early 1980s, North Carolina deaths reached a 20-year low. During economic recovery, deaths go up sharply. North Carolina and the nation are now in a time of economic growth and rising deaths. Belt law effectiveness is therefore being evaluated within the context of a rising death toll. As the impact of the economy on motor vehicle fatalities becomes more clearly documented, such as through the work of Partyka (1984) and Evans and Graham (1988), it should become useful to include these economic factors as control variables in intervention analysis.

6. Finally, there is scientific evidence that drivers with the highest crash risk are least likely to buckle up. The 36 percent who do not buckle up in North Carolina will account for more than 36 percent of total deaths.

The levels of benefit seen and reported here are, in fact, consistent with the factors cited here, though it is also clear from a reading of these factors that the benefit in the United States is only about half what could reasonably be expected if the loopholes were closed and if compliance could be raised to levels more nearly in line with those seen in foreign countries.

Conclusion

Belt laws have made positive contributions to highway safety in the United States, but we have yet to realize the level of compliance and the level of casualty reduction enjoyed by some of the most successful foreign countries. Some of the reasons why that might be so are considered in the final section of this chapter.

Readiness for Seat Belt Laws

Part of the differential success of seat belt laws in the United States and foreign countries may be differences in the degree to which the respective citizens were ready for the mandate. In the United States, widespread organized support for seat belt laws is comparatively recent. Only within the past few years have leading safety organizations, the federal government, and the auto industry endorsed such laws. Soon thereafter several state legislatures began to consider such laws, and a number were passed, sometimes by relatively narrow margins. Thus, in some states the legislature may have been at the very leading edge of public support, or perhaps even ahead of it, as implied by the two recent actions to repeal.

Controversy Regarding Occupant Restraint Issues

If there has been less readiness for the mandate in the United States, the controversy surrounding occupant restraint must surely have played a part. In many other countries, scientists and government officials presented a united front on the subject of occupant restraints, and the thrust was to move in the direction of seat belt laws. In contrast, in the United States, there was significant public controversy over the merits of seat belts versus automatic restraints, and it was often expressed as an "either-or" matter. The issue was a point of dispute by factions within automobile companies, insurance companies, consumer groups, the scientific community, and the government, and was contested between these interests as well. This may have worked to the detriment of acceptance of occupant restraint in *any* form by creating public skepticism on the issue.

Publicity

One difference between the United States and some foreign countries is the degree to which official sources have been able to make use of the media to get and keep the seat belt message before the public. Publicizing belts is more difficult in the United States because of the general prohibition against government-purchased air time. Also, the large number of competing media outlets makes it more difficult to reach a large proportion of the audience.

Many other countries such as Great Britain and Australia have heavily publicized the advantages of seat belts. Public education about the efficacy of belts and advocacy of their use sometimes went on for years before advent of the law itself. For example, Australia has been at the forefront in keeping the safety message before the public. There, the government plays a central role by directly purchasing substantial amounts of media time. Related to the greater official access to TV in foreign countries is the fact that there is less competition for the audience since most other countries have fewer TV channels than does the United States.

Characteristics of the Respective Countries

The success of any attempt to effect widespread change in long-established habitual behaviors, such as the American habit of driving while unrestrained, depends in part on an understanding of the characteristics of the target population. In this part of the discussion consideration is given to such issues as socioeconomic status (SES), literacy, and the homogeneity of the populations. All of these factors may impact upon the successful implementation of seat belt laws.

Socioeconomic differences within the population of the United States could be a relevant factor because of the relatively widespread use of private cars among the poor in America. America is considered the wealthiest large nation on earth, but we may actually have a greater range of socioeconomic differences than exists in other industrialized countries.

Because of the lack of public transportation, and the presence of urban sprawl, which can lead to considerable distance between workplace and dwelling, the motor car is more deeply integrated into the fabric of American society than is the case in many other countries. Thus, for many Americans, a private car is an economic necessity if employment is to be maintained. This is particularly true of low-income individuals whose vocational options are already limited. In other countries, people in the lower SES range might be more likely to use public transportation or to own motorcycles, mopeds, or bicycles rather than cars.

The fact that more low-income individuals in America may be owners or users of private cars is relevant to the issue of seat belt use because of the well-documented fact that seat belt and child restraint use is lowest among persons of lowest SES (Allen and Bergman, 1976; Freedman and Lukin, 1977; Hletko et al., 1983;

Jones, 1979; Kielhorn and Westphal, 1980; and Philpot et al., 1979).

An important part of the final success of seat belt programs in the United States will be related to the ability of public officials to reach lower SES persons and persuade them to become belt users. Experience in other areas of health service delivery suggests this may be a difficult task (Wan, 1977; Bullough, 1972) and that special means must be devised.

Another factor to consider is the fact that the United States is so ethnically diverse. This is important in part because of the link between ethnic minority status and depressed SES. In addition to the economic factors involved, it has been suggested that ethnic minorities may, as a function of a conscious or unconscious need to maintain their ethnic identity, sometimes tend to reject mandates handed down by the "external" majority culture (Baber, 1984).

In such a complex and multiply determined behavior as the wearing of seat belts in compliance to a new law, no single one of the demographic factors noted here could be expected to account for much of the variance seen, but all may enhance or impede the success of the laws to a certain extent.

It should be emphasized that the points presented above should not be construed as an attempt to ascribe to the poor the major responsibility for disappointing use levels and poor compliance with seat belt laws. Such is emphatically not the case. Compliance with seat belt laws is far from perfect in other segments of the population. It still leaves much to be desired among middle-class America!

Concluding Thoughts

The issue of the success of seat belt laws in the United States is not trivial. We have much to gain from the success of such laws. As a stand-alone issue, the enactment of belt laws and the attainment of high compliance therewith can save thousands of lives. Moreover, the success of seat belt laws is not a stand-alone issue. Belt law compliance is related to the success of automatic restraints.

Automatic restraints are now public policy in the United States, and automatic restraints must be installed in 25 percent of this year's car production. Seat belt laws are an important component of the success of our automatic restraint policy. Belt laws will place the sanction of government against the disabling of automatic seat belts in cars so equipped, and in air bag cars, wearing the belt can help to assure that the occupant rides positioned as intended in the air bag design.

Also, some of the findings from analysis of seat belt laws may be repeated when it comes to evaluating the benefits of automatic restraint systems. We need to be prepared for research results which are rather less glowing than the predictions made for automatic restraints. Partly, this is because the automatic restraint devices will, for a long while, tend to be concentrated in the hands of users who are higher in SES and who fall in age groups where crash risk is lower than in the population as a whole. Further, the benefits of automatic restraints will be superimposed on to a time when the mileage death rate is at the historic lowest for the country. It seems likely that by the same token that high-risk drivers are most likely not to comply with belt laws, it may well be that the highest risk drivers will be least likely to drive in cars with automatic restraints, and may be more likely to disable the system or otherwise not take advantage of its benefit characteristics.

Finally, it should be stated again that belt laws have already greatly benefited our citizens. They have already succeeded in reducing fatalities by more than 10,000 and seem likely to have reduced injury by 100,000 or more.

References

ALLEN, D. B., and A. B. BERGMAN. 1976. "Social Learning Approaches to Health Education: Utilization of Infant Auto Restraint Devices." *Pediatrics 58*, no. 3:323–28.

BABER, G. A. 1984. "Patterns of Seat Belt Use Among an Upper Middle Income Black Community with Implications for Public Health Practice." Master's thesis, University of North Carolina, Department of Health Policy and Administration, Chapel Hill.

BOX, G. E. P., and G. M. JENKINS. 1976. *Time Series Analysis: Forecasting and Control*. San Francisco: Holden-Day.

BULLOUGH, B. 1972. "Poverty, Ethnic Identity and Preventive Health Care." *Journal of Health and Social Behavior* 13:347–59.

CAMPBELL, B. J. 1987. *The Relationship of Seat Belt Law Enforcement to Level of Belt Use*. Chapel Hill: Highway Safety Research Center, University of North Carolina.

CAMPBELL, B. J., J. R. STEWART, and FRANCES A. CAMPBELL. 1987. "1985– 1986 Experience with Belt Laws in the United States." Chapel Hill: Highway Safety Research Center, University of North Carolina.

CAMPBELL, B. J., and FRANCES A. CAMPBELL. 1986. *Seat Belt Law Experience in Four Foreign Countries Compared to the United States*. Falls Church, Va.: AAA Foundation for Traffic Safety.

EVANS, W. N., and J. D. GRAHAM, 1988. "Traffic Safety and the Business Cycle," *Alcohol, Drugs, and Driving* 4:31–38.

FREEDMAN, K., and J. LUKIN. 1977. "Occupant Protection for Children: A Survey of Restraint Usage, Attitudes, and Knowledge." New South Wales, Australia: Department of Motor Transport, Traffic Accident Research Unit.

GRIMM, A. C. 1984. "Restraint Use Laws by Country as of August, 1984." *UMTRI Research Review* 15, no. 1. University of Michigan, Ann Arbor.

HEDLUND, J. 1986. "Casualty Reductions: Results from Safety Belt Use Laws." In *Effectiveness of Safety Belt Use Laws*. Washington, D.C.: National Highway Traffic Safety Administration. DOT HS 80 7018.

HLETKO, P. J., J. D. HLETKO, A. M. SHELNESS, and S. S. ROBIN. 1983. "Demographic Predictors of Infant Car Seat Use." *American Journal of Diseases of Children* 137:1061–63.

JONES, D. W. 1979. "An Exploratory Study of Attitudes and Observations on Child Protection in Motor Vehicles." *American Association for Automotive Medicine Journal* 1, no. 4:26–29.

KIELHORN, T. G., and J. WESTPHAL. 1980. "A Study of the Use and Non-use of Child Restraint Devices in Metropolitan Oklahoma." Oklahoma Highway Safety Office.

National Safety Council. 1986. *Accident Facts*, 1986 Edition. Chicago: NSC.

PARTYKA, S. C. 1984. "Simple Models of Fatality Trends Using Employment and Population Data." *Accident Analysis and Prevention* 16:211–222.

PHILPOT, J. W., K. W. HEATHINGTON, R. L. PERRY, and E. C. HUGHES. 1979. "The Use of Child Passenger Safety Devices in Tennessee." Knoxville: The University of Tennessee.

WAGENAAR, A. C., R. G. MAYBEE, and K. P. SULLIVAN. 1987. "Michigan's Compulsory Restraint Use Policies: Effects on Injuries and Deaths." Ann Arbor: University of Michigan Transportation Research Institute, UMTRI 87-10.

———. In press. "Mandatory Seat Belt Laws in Eight States: A Time-series Analysis." *Journal of Safety Research*.

WAN, T. 1977. "The Differential Use of Health Services: A Minority Perspective." *Urban Health* 6:48–52.

WILLIAMS, A. F., D. F. PREUSSER, R. D. BLOMBERG, and A. K. LUND. 1986. "Results of a Seat Belt Use Law Enforcement and Publicity Campaign in Elmira, N.Y." Washington D.C.: Insurance Institute for Highway Safety.

Chapter 3

MANDATORY SEAT BELT USE LAWS AND OCCUPANT CRASH PROTECTION IN THE UNITED STATES: PRESENT STATUS AND FUTURE PROSPECTS

by Allan F. Williams and
Adrian K. Lund

The Problem

In the 10-year period from 1975 to 1984, about 225,000 car drivers and right front seat passengers were killed in motor vehicle crashes in the United States (NHTSA, 1975–1984). If all these occupants had been wearing seat belts, almost 100,000 would not have died. Belts, if worn, restrain occupants so that they stay inside the vehicle and so that their contact with harmful interior structures is reduced or eliminated. Most cars on the road during this time were equipped with manual seat belts; therefore, using belts was a readily available option. However, universal application of this preventive action requires that each person fasten a seat belt on each car trip. In fact, voluntary belt use in the United States has

This work was supported by the Insurance Institute for Highway Safety. The assistance of Michele Fields, Steve Oesch, and Sharon Rasmussen is gratefully acknowledged.

51

always been unusual behavior. During the 1975–1984 period, use rates by drivers ranged between 10 and 18 percent; belt use by right front passengers was somewhat lower (NHTSA, 1978; 1984). The few people who choose to wear belts tend to be low-risk drivers; thus, belt use by occupants involved in crashes—the population of concern—is lower yet (Deutsch, Sameth, and Akinyemi, 1980; Evans and Wasielewski, 1983). In addition, when belt users are in crashes, their crashes tend to be less severe, as measured by vehicle damage scales, than crashes of nonusers (NHTSA, 1985).

Failure of Educational Programs

Many types of educational and persuasive techniques have been tried in an effort to get more people to use belts, but the effect of those efforts has been slight or nil (Kelley and Robertson, 1978; Fisher, 1980). Many nonusers say they believe belts are effective and agree that it makes sense to wear them (Fhaner and Hane, 1972), but the crash risk per person per trip is extremely low, and most people have chosen to travel unbelted. In fact, seat belt use actually decreased during the late 1970s, a period in which various preventive health actions related to nutrition, physical activity, and smoking were being performed in increasing numbers by the U.S. population (Williams, 1982). Seat belt education may have some positive benefits in creating a climate that facilitates passage of belt use laws, but it has not worked to increase seat belt use directly in the United States or in other countries (Fisher, 1980).

Belt Use Incentives

Economic incentives have been used with some success as a means of increasing seat belt use, but their application is limited. Programs based on rewarding people for using seat belts by giving them t-shirts, gift certificates, or the like have successfully increased usage, but when the rewards are discontinued, belt use declines (Campbell, Hunter, and Gemming, 1983; Geller, Johnson, and Pelton, 1982). Employer-sponsored incentive programs may be the best mechanism for increasing and maintaining use because an employer can sustain rewards over time in the same population. Some employer programs have been successful in this regard (Streff and Geller, 1986). It has been suggested that automobile insurance discounts could be used as an incentive to increase use. However, a recent review of insurance incentives noted that less than 20 percent of the total automobile coverage and premium lends itself to a reduction due to the insured's seat belt use and concluded that "It is unlikely that any insurance company will offer substantial up-front incentives for those who claim to be belt wearers because there are serious problems with trusting the insureds to wear belts and with denying payments to insureds who are injured while not wearing belts" (NHTSA, 1983). Insurance rewards based on increased compensation payments for clients injured or killed in a motor vehicle crash have been evaluated and found to be ineffective in increasing belt use (Robertson, 1984). Negative incentives, in the form of decreased damage payments for crash injuries if not wearing a belt, have not been evaluated but are also unlikely to be effective in increasing use. Many states specifically prohibit or substantially limit the introduction of evidence on belt use for the purpose of reducing damages awarded in civil suits involving vehicle crashes (Westenberg, 1983).

Belt Use Laws in Other Countries

To improve seat belt use rates, about 30 countries throughout the world enacted laws during the 1970s and early 1980s requiring motorists to use seat belts. There is variation in the effectiveness of these laws; use rates ranging from as low as 3 percent to as high as over 90 percent have been reported. Many of the laws have succeeded in raising use rates to 50 percent or greater and reducing fatalities and serious injuries somewhat. The first seat belt use law was enacted in Victoria, Australia, in 1970; Australia has also been among the most successful countries in achieving high usage rates.

The U.S. Approach

FMVSS 208 History. Although the majority of state legislatures in the United States considered seat belt use legislation during the 1970s, no belt use laws were passed. Educational programs remained the primary means of attempting to increase belt use, and usage remained low.

The infrequent use of manual belts had been anticipated in the United States before belts were required to be installed in all new cars and their lack of use became apparent. In early 1967, William Haddon, Jr., administrator of the National Traffic Safety Agency and the National Highway Safety Bureau (predecessors of the National Highway Traffic Safety Administration [NHTSA]), told the Senate Commerce Committee that automatic (or passive) restraints—such as air bags—would be mandated as soon as the

technology permitted. Automatic restraints are intended to work
without any action being required by occupants. According to
Haddon, "We would far prefer to adopt only standards that pose
no problem to anyone and that do not require any active cooperation on the part of the user. This is the approach, after all, which
has been used in public health going back 50 and 100 years with
such programs as pasteurization of milk, chlorination of water
supplies, and so forth" (Haddon, 1967).

Rule making on automatic restraints was begun in 1969. In 1970
a notice of proposed rule making was issued on Federal Motor
Vehicle Safety Standard (FMVSS) 208, Occupant Crash Protection,
requiring passenger cars manufactured after January 1, 1973 to be
equipped with automatic restraints. The automatic restraint provisions of FMVSS 208 were debated at length during the next
decade, the period during which most other industrialized countries of the world were enacting seat belt use laws; these provisions
of standard 208 were delayed or altered several times. Automobile
manufacturers generally opposed these provisions, which were
vigorously supported by public health groups. In 1981 the standard
was canceled by NHTSA; in 1982 NHTSA was ordered by the
courts to reconsider this decision. In October 1983 NHTSA issued
a notice of proposed rule making that put forth various options,
including reinstatement of the standard, amending the standard,
and total rescission. Hearings were conducted later that year.

Child Restraint Laws. Although no seat belt use laws were
passed in the United States in the 1970s and early 1980s, states—
beginning with Tennessee in 1978—initiated laws requiring restraints to be used for infants and young children. The ground-
breaking effort in Tennessee was led by the state's pediatricians, in
particular Dr. Robert Sanders. By mid-1985, all 50 states and the
District of Columbia had enacted child restraint laws, many of
which allowed use of seat belts as an alternative to special child
restraint devices. A logical next step was to extend these laws to
other ages, which was first done in New York, a state that histori-
cally has been a leader in applying policies to reduce motor vehicle
injuries. New York issued a regulation in 1983 that required seat
belt use by learners' permit holders. Following this regulation, a
law requiring belt use by junior licensees and probationary license
holders was passed and then was superseded by another law
requiring belt use by all front seat occupants beginning in December 1984.

FMVSS 208 Final Rule. After New York's belt use law was
passed, a final rule on FMVSS 208 was issued. Under this rule,
automobile manufacturers were again required to install automatic

restraints in all new cars by the 1990 model year, starting with 10 percent in 1987, then 25 percent in 1988, and 40 percent in 1989. However, if states comprising two-thirds of the nation's population pass seat belt use laws meeting certain minimum criteria by 1989, the automatic restraint requirements will be rescinded. These criteria include:

- Requiring proper seat belt use by drivers and front seat passengers of passenger cars required by federal regulation to be equipped with seat belts.
- Issuing no waivers except for medical reasons.
- Providing a minimum $25 fine for violations.
- Requiring that violations of the law may be used in mitigating damages sought by that person in litigation to recover damages for crash injuries.
- Establishing prevention and education programs to encourage compliance with the laws (49 C.F.R.).

Passage of State Seat Belt Laws

Since the 1984 rule, seat belt use laws have proliferated. The laws have been spurred in large part by a multimillion dollar lobbying campaign sponsored by U.S. automobile manufacturers. As of late 1987, more than 60 percent of the states had such laws, and about 80 percent of the population was covered by them. However, the automatic restraint provisions of FMVSS 208 are currently in effect. As noted by the U.S. Court of Appeals in a 1986 decision in which it refused to rule on a suit challenging the legality of the FMVSS rescission provisions of the final rule, it is unlikely that the automatic restraint requirements will be rescinded because virtually none of the first 20 belt use laws enacted met the criteria specified in the rule (*State Farm* v. *Dole,* 1986).

The states, effective dates of the laws, and penalty and enforcement provisions are provided in Table 3–1. There is variation in the laws in terms of the criteria specified by NHTSA; they also differ in a way not anticipated by the rule making. Only nine of the states permit motorists to be stopped or cited for a seat belt law violation alone (primary enforcement). In the other states, a vehicle must first be stopped or cited for some other traffic offense (secondary enforcement). The United States is unusual in this respect; less than 25 percent of the world's jurisdictions with seat belt use laws do not allow primary enforcement (NHTSA, 1986). Permissible fines for belt use law violations range from nothing (Minnesota) to up to $50 (New Mexico, New York, Oregon, Texas).

Table 3–1   U.S. Seat Belt Laws, as of December 1, 1987

State	Effective Date	Penalty	Enforcement Provision*
New York	Dec. 1984	Up to $50	Primary
New Jersey	March 1985	$20	Secondary
Illinois	July 1985	Up to $25	Secondary
Michigan	July 1985	$25	Secondary
Missouri	Sept. 1985	Up to $10	Secondary
Texas	Sept. 1985	$25–$50	Primary
North Carolina	Oct. 1985	$25	Primary
District of Columbia	Dec. 1985	Up to $15	Secondary
Hawaii	Dec. 1985	$15	Primary
California	Jan. 1986	Up to $20 for first offense; up to $50 for second offense	Secondary
Connecticut	Jan. 1986	$15	Primary
New Mexico	Jan. 1986	$25–$50	Primary
Tennessee	April 1986	$25 for second offense	Secondary
Utah	April 1986	$10	Secondary
Ohio	May 1986	Driver, $20; passenger, $10	Secondary
Washington	June 1986	$20	Secondary
Florida	July 1986	$20	Secondary
Idaho	July 1986	Up to $5	Secondary
Iowa	July 1986	$10	Primary
Kansas	July 1986	Up to $10	Secondary
Louisiana	July 1986	$25	Secondary
Maryland	July 1986	Up to $25	Secondary
Minnesota	August 1986	No fine	Primary
Oklahoma	Feb. 1987	$25	Secondary
Colorado	July 1987	$10	Secondary
Indiana	July 1987	Up to $25	Secondary
Nevada	July 1987	Up to $25	Secondary
Oregon	Sept. 1987	Up to $50	Primary
Pennsylvania	Nov. 1987	$10	Secondary
Wisconsin	Dec. 1987	$10	Secondary
Montana	Jan. 1988	$20	Secondary
Virginia	Jan. 1988	$25	Secondary
Repealed:			
Nebraska	Sept. 1985 to Dec. 1986	$25	Secondary
Massachusetts	Jan. 1986 to Dec. 1986	$15	Secondary

*Primary enforcement: a police officer can stop a motorist simply for failure to wear a seat belt; secondary enforcement: a vehicle must first be stopped for some other traffic offense before a ticket may be given for not wearing a seat belt.

Effects of the Laws on Fatalities and Injuries

At this date many of the laws are still relatively new; most of them have been in effect for less than two years. Nevertheless, the laws, especially the initial ones, have been studied by many investigators and their effects on belt use rates and on injuries and fatalities can be estimated with some confidence. The following summary statements can be made about the effects of the laws:

1. Use rates increased in states that passed laws, from very low levels before the laws went into effect to between 40 and 60 percent right after (Williams, Wells, and Lund, 1987).

2. The typical pattern is that the highest use rates are achieved immediately after the laws go into force—that is, in the first month—followed by declines within a few months and eventual stabilization. Data from Michigan, displayed in Figure 3–1, illustrate this phenomenon (Wagenaar, Molnar, and Businski, 1987).

3. There are substantial state-to-state variations in use rates. The Insurance Institute for Highway Safety has carried out observational surveys of belt use in several states. Figures 3–2 to 3–5 show belt use rates over time in large cities of four states that account for 30 percent of the population of the United States. These rates are based on large numbers of observations (typically

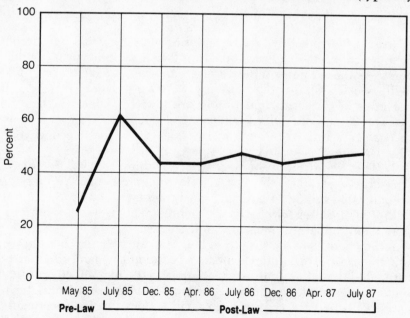

Figure 3-1 Belt Use by Front Seat Occupants in Michigan.

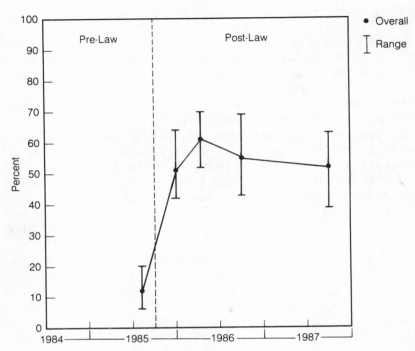

Figure 3-2   Belt Use by Front Seat Occupants in Texas (Large Cities).

at least 1,000 per city per observation period), with 95 percent confidence intervals of plus or minus 2 to 3 percent for individual cities. As these figures indicate, use rates in Texas have been quite high; two years after the law they were 52 percent. In contrast, use rates in California and Illinois are low. In California, the use rate was 37 percent in large cities one year after the law; in Illinois, the use rate was 33 percent at the end of the law's second year. The use rate in New York was 44 percent after two years.

4. The variation in experience for different states relates strongly to whether the law can be enforced on a primary or secondary basis and to how vigorously the law is enforced (Campbell, 1987). States with primary enforcement provisions have experienced the largest increases in use rates.

If the changes in belt use from before to after the law are known, the theoretical maximum expected reduction in fatalities can be estimated based on the known injury-reducing effectiveness of belts. For example, an increase from 15 to 45 percent translates to about a 15 percent reduction in fatalities of front seat occupants. The theoretical fatality reduction is computed by the formula $R = [(AE - BE)/(1 - BE)]*100$, where R is the percent reduction in

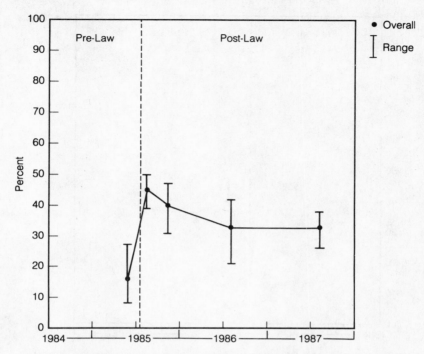

Figure 3-3   Belt Use by Front Seat Occupants in Illinois (Large Cities).

fatalities, *A* is the proportion using belts after the law, *B* is the proportion using belts prelaw, and *E* is the proportional reduction in the likelihood of fatality in a crash (0.45) (49 C.F.R. 571.208). However, this assumes that belt use rates achieved in daily traffic are equal to those in the crash population, and typically this is not the case. Motorists with higher crash or injury risks (e.g., males, teenagers, speeders) are also less likely than other drivers to comply with belt use laws (Williams, Wells, and Lund, 1987; Preusser, Williams, and Lund, 1987; Preusser et al., 1987). Drinking drivers, who are major contributors to fatal and serious injury crashes, are less likely than others to comply with belt use laws (Ministry of Transportation and Communications, 1979). Drivers leaving bars on weekend nights in New York State were found to wear belts much less often than other nighttime drivers (Preusser, Williams, and Lund, 1986). The result is that fatality reductions are usually less than would be expected based on results from surveys of daily traffic; this has been the experience of countries around the world with belt use laws (Williams and O'Neill, 1979; Hurst, 1979). Figure 3–6 illustrates this phenomenon in the United States.

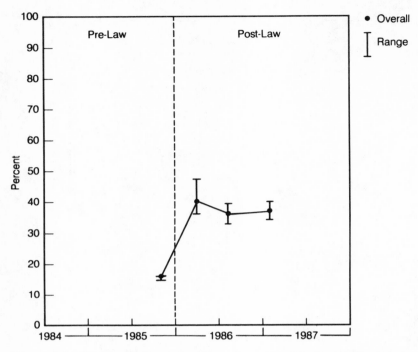

Figure 3-4 Belt Use by Front Seat Occupants in California (Large Cities).

Table 3–2 summarizes the results of multistate evaluations of fatality changes resulting from belt use laws. These five studies indicate that the estimated reductions in fatalities and injuries resulting from the laws are in the range of 5 to 15 percent, and they are generally on the lower end of this range. As expected, when individual states are examined, states with higher use rates generally have greater fatality decreases; the fatality reduction in Texas, for example, was estimated at 19 percent (Campbell, Stewart, and Campbell, 1987). Consistent with the decline in use rates experienced during the postlaw periods by most states, declines in fatality reductions over time have also been reported (Hoxie and Skinner, 1987).

Future Prospects

Based primarily on these studies, the best current estimate is that states with laws will experience, on average, an annual reduction in occupant fatalities of 5 to 10 percent. If this is the case, the main uncertainty in terms of future prospects is how many more states

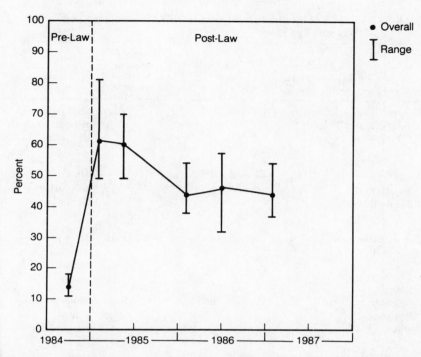

Figure 3-5 Belt Use by Front Seat Occupants in New York State (Large Cities).

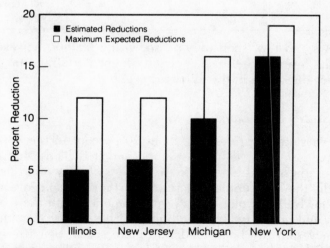

Figure 3-6 Estimated Reductions in Front Seat Occupant Fatalities Compared with Maximum Reductions Expected from Changes in Seat Belt Use.

Table 3–2   Results of Multistate Studies of Fatality Changes Associated with
Seat Belt Use Laws

Author (year)	No. of States Studied	Post-Law Time Period Covered	Average or Range of Fatality Change (%)	Methods Employed
Campbell and Campbell (1986)	8	through 1985	− 10	Time series— comparison with all nonlaw states
Campbell, Stewart, and Campbell (1987)	25	through 1986	− 7	Time series— comparison with all nonlaw states
Lund, Zador, and Pollner (1987)	4	through 1985	− 5 to − 16	Time series— regional comparison states
Wagenaar, Maybec and Sullivan (1987)	8	through 1985	− 9	Time series— paired comparison states
Hoxie and Skinner (1987)	18	though June 1986	− 6	Cross-sectional time series— comparison with all nonlaw states

pass laws and how soon they do so. Other factors, however, will affect the future of belt use laws and occupant restraint in general; these are discussed in the following section.

More States with Laws

Nineteen states representing about 20 percent of the population still have not enacted belt use laws, and it is likely that at least some of these states will do so. The states without laws are generally the less populous states, so further gains in coverage will come slowly. It is notable that, in conjunction with the legislative activity and publicity about belt use that has occurred in all states, there have already been moderate increases in belt use in some cities without laws (NHTSA, 1987a). About nine years elapsed between the time the first and the fiftieth states passed child restraint laws; it has been only a little over three years since New

York State enacted the first belt use law. It is, of course, possible that the greater resistance to belt use legislation that presumably exists in states without laws than in the states that earlier enacted laws will be reflected in lower postlaw use rates.

There is also the possibility that states with laws will repeal them. Massachusetts and Nebraska have already done so via binding referenda, and use rates have declined substantially from 40 to 28 percent in Nebraska (J. B. Williams, 1987) and from 37 to 24 percent in Massachusetts (Hingson et al., 1987). Survey data collected in Massachusetts indicated that invasion of personal liberty and the perceived ineffectiveness of the law were major issues for those voting for repeal (Hingson et al., 1987). Repeal activity has also taken place in other states, and Oregon will have a binding referendum on its belt use law in November 1988. In addition, the laws in Missouri and Michigan are written so that they are to be rescinded in 1989 if the automatic restraint provisions of FMVSS 208 become effective. A "sunset" clause provides that the Tennessee law is automatically repealed effective June 30, 1990 unless legislation is enacted to extend it; if Tennessee's law is not counted by NHTSA as part of the population covered by belt laws, it can be rescinded earlier. The Colorado belt law is repealed effective July 1, 1989 unless Colorado fatality statistics show improvement in 1988. The North Carolina law will be rescinded if the U.S. Department of Transportation decides that the law does not comply with its minimum criteria for effective mandatory use laws. Thus the progression toward the remainder of the population being covered by belt use laws is not altogether certain.

Changes in Existing Laws

Few changes have been made in the belt use laws that have been enacted since 1984. Illinois in 1987 changed its laws so that it specifically calls for secondary enforcement. In other states, such as California, there has been legislative debate about strengthening the law by changing a secondary enforcement provision to primary.

Most of the laws have gaps in their coverage—that is, some occupants of motor vehicles in which belts are available are not required to use them. Only California, Montana, Nevada, Washington, and Wisconsin require all rear seat occupants to use seat belts. Several states limit the types of vehicles covered. For example, Louisiana, New Mexico, and Oklahoma exclude pickup trucks from coverage; yet, occupants of pickup trucks comprised about 30 percent of occupant deaths in these states prior to the laws (NHTSA, 1975–1984).

The original child restraint laws also had many gaps in coverage such that about 20 percent of the children who had been killed in crashes before the laws went into effect would not have been required to be restrained under the law (Teret et al., 1986). Subsequent law changes have removed some of these gaps in child restraint law coverage. The potential for similar changes in regard to belt use laws is also present.

Possible Higher Use Rates in States with Laws

In most states with laws, the majority of motorists do not use seat belts; several states have reported use rates in the range of 25 to 35 percent (Campbell, Stewart, and Campbell, 1987). Although an improvement over prelaw rates, these use rates limit the effects of the laws. There is large variation in belt use in the states, but even in the most successful states use rates are considerably lower than in countries such as Australia, West Germany, and the United Kingdom, where use rates of 90 percent or greater prevail. When seat belt laws are being debated in this country, it was believed that what happened in some Canadian provinces when they passed belt use laws might be most indicative of what would happen in the United States. The early experience of the Canadian provinces that enacted seat belt laws in the 1970s is quite similar to the early experience in the United States. Several of the provinces experienced sharp increases in initial use rates, followed by declines within a few months. In 1980, shoulder belt use rates were 49 percent in British Columbia, 44 percent in Ontario, and 39 percent in Quebec (Transport Canada, 1987).

Historical, cultural, and demographic explanations for the less successful experience with belt use laws in the United States (and Canada), compared to Europe and Australia (Campbell and Campbell, 1986), have been discussed, but these explanations provide little guidance for increasing belt use. Rather, the most fruitful approach has focused on improving enforcement of the laws. Experience worldwide has indicated that enforcement, or at least perceived enforcement, of belt use laws is the key factor in achieving and maintaining high belt use rates. Officials in several Canadian provinces recognized that seat belts use laws could be more successful in reducing fatalities and initiated programs designed to provide stepped-up enforcement of the laws. These programs, which involved intensified enforcement accompanied by heightened publicity, successfully increased use rates. For example, a one-month program in Ottawa, Ontario, increased belt use from 58 percent before the program to 80 percent right after;

two years later belt use was still 66 percent (Jonah, Dawson, and Smith, 1982). Over this period belt use dropped from 54 to 43 percent in Kingston, Ontario, a comparison city without a program. Largely as a result of increased enforcement and publicity efforts, belt use has increased in Canadian provinces during the 1980s (Figure 3–7). In 1986 belt use was 78 percent in British Columbia, 66 percent in Ontario, and 68 percent in Quebec. These rates are higher than current belt use rates in *any* of the American states with laws.

A three-week enforcement/publicity campaign, similar to those in Canada, was conducted in November 1985 in Elmira, New York, a city of about 35,000 people (Williams et al., 1987a). This program increased belt use from 49 to 77 percent right after the program; four months later belt use was 66 percent. A subsequent reminder campaign conducted in Elmira in the spring of 1986 increased use to 80 percent; use declined to 69 percent four months later and 60 percent eight months later (Williams et al., 1987b). Throughout these periods, belt use in Glens Falls, a comparison community, remained stable at just over 40 percent. Successful belt use law enforcement/publicity programs have also been run in other New York communities (NHTSA, 1987b).

New York's law allows primary enforcement, which makes enforcement campaigns more straightforward to conduct. An enforce-

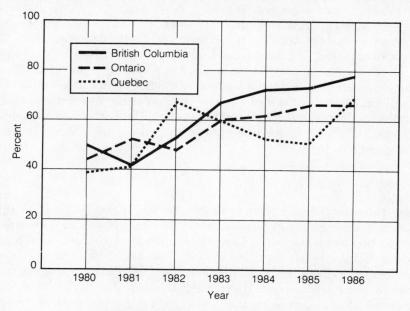

Figure 3-7 Driver Belt Use in Three Canadian Provinces.

ment campaign conducted in Modesto, California, confirmed that enforcement campaigns in states with secondary enforcement will require more effort to achieve the same levels of usage as in states with primary enforcement. Nevertheless, belt use increased from 33 to 57 percent in the Modesto program, indicating that such programs can also successfully increase belt use even in secondary enforcement states such as California (Stuster and Lund, 1987).

Thus in the United States, as in Canada, publicly visible enforcement campaigns can substantially increase compliance with belt use laws. This has been shown to be the case in other countries as well. For example, a publicity/enforcement campaign conducted in 1984 in the Netherlands succeeded in raising use rates by 15 to 25 percentage points (Gundy, 1987). Although some countries have apparently achieved high usage rates without strong enforcement of the laws, in the United States the amount of enforcement is a strong correlate of belt use. The likely level of compliance that can be achieved and the levels of enforcement that police and community leaders judge as politically desirable and feasible in the United States are yet to be determined.

Now that many states have passed laws and their initial effects are known, the realization has come that it is not sufficient simply to pass a belt use law; efforts have to be made after the law goes into force to maximize its effects. This realization was formalized in 1987 when a consortium of safety, government, and auto industry organizations met and agreed to work to increase belt use rates in the United States to 70 percent by 1990 (Bronrott, 1987). Specifically, the "Reston Accord" calls on every state to enact a belt use law and to carry out education and enforcement programs. Evidence from the Canadian provinces suggests that belt use rates of about 70 percent are possible with increased enforcement and publicity. Whether the substantial and continuing efforts needed to accomplish this goal will be put forth in the United States is not known at this time.

Automatic Restraints

The provision of automatic restraints in accordance with FMVSS 208 will have an effect on mandatory belt use laws and occupant protection. The two ways the injury criteria of the standard are being met are by air bags that inflate automatically from inside the steering wheel or dashboard in crashes and by seat belts that fasten around occupants when they enter the car. In 1987 about 90 percent of the cars with automatic restraints had belt systems rather than air bags. Most manufacturers will also meet the 25 percent requirement in 1988 cars with automatic belts. These cars represent only a small fraction of all the cars presently on the road, but automatic belts should help to increase use rates both in states with and without laws. However, this depends on the type of automatic belt provided. The automatic belts that are being offered differ in ease of use and in the ease and manner in which they can be detached or disabled. A recent observational survey conducted in suburban Washington, D.C., Chicago, Los Angeles, and Philadelphia indicated that some manufacturers have been more successful than others in providing automatic belt systems that result in high use and increased injury protection (Williams et al., 1987c). In this study, use of automatic belts was compared with use of manual belts in late model cars at the same make and model (Table 3–3).

The automatic belts provided by Ford and Toyota (motorized, nondetachable shoulder belt), Nissan (motorized, detachable shoulder belt), and VW (nonmotorized, detachable shoulder belt with ignition interlock) increased use rates to about 90 percent. This occurred in both law and nonlaw areas and, in fact, increases tended to be greater in nonlaw areas because of lower manual belt use rates. For example, in Philadelphia (no law) shoulder belt use in Ford cars was 39 percent in manual belt cars and 88 percent in automatic belt cars; in Los Angeles (law) manual and automatic

Table 3–3 Shoulder Belt Use by Front Seat Occupants in Late Model Cars with Manual or Automatic Belt Systems

Manufacturer and Belt Use		Percent (Number)	
		Law[a]	No Law[b]
Chrysler:	Manual	71 (136)	47 (129)
	Automatic	53 (45)	36 (136)
Ford:	Manual	55 (864)	46 (484)
	Automatic	85 (350)	89 (190)
GM:	Manual	59 (2024)	48 (1158)
	Automatic	68 (710)	53 (238)
Nissan:	Manual	65 (442)	58 (255)
	Automatic	89 (261)	86 (127)
Toyota:	Manual	74 (420)	73 (207)
	Automatic	96 (857)	98 (300)
VW:	Manual	65 (615)	63 (381)
	Automatic	89 (73)	89 (61)

[a]Chicago, Los Angeles, and Maryland suburbs of Washington, D.C.
[b]Philadelphia and Virginia suburbs of Washington, D.C.

shoulder belt use rates in Ford cars were 59 and 87 percent, respectively.

In GM cars (detachable lap and shoulder belt) there were smaller but statistically significant increases in belt use that occurred both in law and nonlaw areas. For example, manual shoulder belt use was 41 percent in Philadelphia, and automatic shoulder belt use 47 percent; in Los Angeles, manual and automatic shoulder belt use rates were 63 and 77 percent, respectively. GM cars with automatic belts have a three-point lap and shoulder belt, so that the observed increases in use were for both lap and shoulder belts.

Chrysler provides a detachable, nonmotorized automatic shoulder belt system that actually decreases use in comparison to usage in late-model Chrysler cars equipped with manual belts. However, in general, the automatic belts presently provided by manufacturers do serve to increase belt use rates.

Air Bags

All the domestic manufacturers have made commitments to air bag technology, and the prospects are good that by the early 1990s the majority of new cars manufactured in the United States will have at least driver-side air bags. The situation in regard to occupant protection then changes, because air bags will most likely be offered along with manual lap and shoulder belts, thus introducing the possibility of their combined protection.

The debate about automatic restraints that took place during the 1970s probably hindered efforts to get belt use laws passed by posing belt use laws and air bags as alternatives, and, in fact, that debate was formalized as laws versus air bags in the FMVSS 208 final rule. Interestingly, there is now the possibility that many of the future cars in the United States will have two complementary systems that could greatly enhance crash protection. Air bags provide a baseline of protection to those car occupants who do not comply with belt use laws and add to the protection of those who do use belts, particularly by preventing head and face contacts with interior structures in high-speed frontal collisions.

In terms of providing maximum crash protection, the combination of seat belts and air bags provides the most effective restraint system available today. Table 3–4 shows the estimated number of lives that could be saved in the United States in 1990 with varying levels of belt use in crashes, as estimated from figures provided by the Department of Transportation (49 C.F.R. 571.208). For example, with a 50 percent use rate in crashes, the lives saved are approximately doubled with the addition of air bags. The number

Table 3–4 Projected Lives Saved in 1990 by Lap/Shoulder Belts and Air Bags

% Belt Usage Rate	Lives Saved		
	Lap/Shoulder Belt	Lap/Shoulder Belt Plus Air Bag	Difference
0	0	7,540	7,540
20	2,310	8,590	6,280
40	4,610	9,640	5,030
50	5,770	10,150	4,380
70	8,080	11,230	3,150
90	10,380	12,260	1,880

Note: Based on DOT estimates of driver and right front seat fatal injuries in 1990 (25,640 absent restraints) and the effectiveness of occupant restraint systems; projections rounded to nearest 10.

of serious injuries prevented would also be more than doubled. A 50 percent belt use rate in crashes implies a use rate in daily traffic substantially greater than 50 percent; this is an optimistic but possible scenario if all states enacted belt use laws and enforced them. Even if a 70 percent rate in crashes were somehow achieved, the addition of air bags would save many additional lives. The implicit assumption in the presentation of the data in Table 3–4 is that when air bags are provided, manual lap and shoulder belts will be used at the same rate as in the absence of the air bags. That may not be true, but even if their use is lower, the addition of air bags would markedly reduce deaths. Air bags alone, without *any* use of seat belts, would prevent an estimated 7,540 deaths.

The most optimistic scenario for the future is most or all states with belt use laws, more states with primary enforcement laws, widespread efforts to maximize belt usage, and the combination of successful belt use laws with widespread availability of air bags. The United States lagged behind much of the rest of the world in the 1970s and early 1980s in terms of advancing occupant restraint; in the 1990s there is the possibility it will surpass many countries in the crash protection its car occupants receive from restraints.

References

BRONROTT, B. 1987. "New Nationwide Effort Launched to Boost Safety Belt Use." Washington, D.C.: National Association of Governor's Highway Safety Representatives.

CAMPBELL, B. J. 1987. "The Relationship of Seat Belt Law Enforcement to Level of Belt Use." Chapel Hill, N.C.: University of North Carolina Highway Safety Research Center.

CAMPBELL, B. J., and F. A. CAMPBELL 1986. "Seat Belt Law in Experience in Four Foreign Countries Compared to the United States." Falls Church, Va.: AAA Foundation for Traffic Safety.

CAMPBELL, B. J., W. HUNTER, and M. GEMMING. 1983. "Seat Belts Pay Off: A Communitywide Research/Public Service Project Designed to Increase Use of Lap and Shoulder Belts. Interim Report." Chapel Hill, N.C.: University of North Carolina, Highway Safety Research Center.

CAMPBELL, B. J., J. R. STEWART, and F. A. CAMPBELL. 1987. "1985–1986 Experience with Belt Use Laws in the United States." Chapel Hill, N.C.: University of North Carolina, Highway Safety Research Center.

DEUTSCH, D., S. SAMETH, and J. AKINYEMI. "Seat Belt Usage and Risk-taking Behavior at Two Major Intersections." *24th Annual Proceedings of the American Association for Automotive Medicine*. Morton Grove, Ill., pp. 415–21.

EVANS, L., and P. WASIELEWSKI. 1983. "Risky Driving Related to Driver and Vehicle Characteristics." *Accident Analysis and Prevention* 15:121–36.

FHANER, G., and M. HANE. 1972. "Seat Belts: Factors Influencing Their Use." *Accident Analysis & Prevention* 5:27–43.

FISHER, F. B., JR. "Effectiveness of Safety Belt Usage Laws." Washington, D.C.: National Highway Safety Administration, U.S. Department of Transportation.

GELLER, E. S., E. P. JOHNSON, and S. L. PELTON. 1982. "Community-Based Interventions for Encouraging Safety Belt Use." *American Journal of Community Psychology* 10:183–95.

GUNDY, C. M. 1987. The Effectiveness of a Combination of Police Enforcement and Public Information for Improving Seat Belt Use." Presented at Second International Conference on Road Safety. Insurance for Road Safety Research (SWOV), The Netherlands.

HADDON, WILLIAM, JR. 1967. Statement before the Committee on Commerce, United States Senate, on implementation of the National Traffic and Motor Vehicle Safety Act of 1966, March 20, 1967. Washington, D.C.: U.S. Government Printing Office, 55–63.

HINGSON, R., S. M. LEVENSON, T. HEEREN, T. MANGIONE, C. RODGERS, T. SCHIAVONNE, and R. HERTZ. 1987. "Repeal of the Massachusetts Seat Belt Law." *American Journal of Public Health,* in press.

HOXIE, P., and D. SKINNER, 1987. "Fatality Reductions from Mandatory Seatbelt Usage Laws." Cambridge, Mass.: Transportation Systems Center.

HURST, P. M. 1979. "Compulsory Seat Belt Use: Further Interference." *Accident Analysis & Prevention* 11:27–34.

JONAH, B. A., N. E. DAWSON, and G. A. SMITH. 1982. "Effects of a Selective Traffic Enforcement Program on Seat Belt Usage." *Journal of Applied Psychology* 67:89–96.

KELLEY, B., and L. S. ROBERTSON. 1978. Statement Before the Subcommittee on Investigations and Review, House Committee on Public Works and Transportation. Hearings on Safety Belt Usage, June 7, Insurance Institute for Highway Safety, Washington. D.C.

LUND, A. K., P. L. ZADOR, and J. POLLNER. 1987. "Motor Vehicle Occupant Fatalities in Four States with Seat Belt Use Laws." SAE Technical Paper 870224. Warrendale, Penn.: Society of Automotive Engineers.

Ministry of Transportation and Communications. 1979. *The 1979 Ontario Road-side BAC Summary Report*. Ottawa, Ontario: The Ministry.

National Highway Traffic Safety Administration (NHTSA). 1975–1984. *Fatal Accident Reporting System*. Washington, D.C.: U.S. Department of Transportation.

———. 1978. *Safety Belt Usage: Survey of the Traffic Population*. Washington, D.C.: U.S. Department of Transportation.

———. 1983. *Assessment of Insurance Incentives for Safety Belt Usage*. Washington, D.C.: U.S. Department of Transportation.

———. 1984. *Restraint System Usage in the Traffic Population*. Washington, D.C.: U.S. Department of Transportation.

———. 1985. *National Accident Sampling System*. Washington, D.C.: U.S. Department of Transportation.

———. 1986. *Effectiveness of Safety Belt Use Laws: A Mutlinational Examination*. Washington, D.C.: U.S. Department of Transportation.

———. 1987a. *Restraint System Usage in the Traffic Population*. Washington, D.C.: U.S. Department of Transportation.

———. 1987b. *Selective Traffic Enforcement Program for Occupant Restraints*. Washington, D.C.: U.S. Department of Transportation.

PREUSSER, D. F., A. K. LUND, A. F. WILLIAMS, and R. D. BLOMBERG. 1987. "Belt Use by High Risk Drivers Before and After New York's Seat Belt Use Law." *Accident Analysis & Prevention,* in press.

PREUSSER, D. F., A. F. WILLIAMS, and A. K. LUND. 1986. "Seat Belt Use Among New York Bar Patrons." *Journal of Public Health Policy* 7, no. 4:470–79.

———. 1987. "The Effect of New York's Seat Belt Use Law on Teenage Drivers." *Accident Analysis & Prevention* 19, no.2:73–80.

ROBERTSON, L. S. 1984. "Insurance Incentives and Seat Belt Use." *American Journal of Public Health* 74, no. 10:1157–58.

State Farm v. Dole, 802 F. 2d 474, 480–81 (D.C. Cir. 1986).

STREFF, F. M., and E. S. GELLER. 1986. "Strategies for Motivating Safety Belt Use: The Application of Applied Behavior Analysis." *Health Education Research, Theory and Practice* 1:47–59.

STUSTER, J. W., and A. K. LUND. 1987. "Special Publicity and Enforcement of California's Belt Use Law: Making a 'Secondary' Law Work." Washington, D.C.: Insurance Institute for Highway Safety.

TERET, S. P., A. S. JONES, A. F. WILLIAMS, and J. K. WELLS. "Child Restraint Laws: An Analysis of Gaps in Coverage." *American Journal of Public Health* 76, no.1:31–34.

Transport Canada. 1987. *Estimates of Shoulder Seat Belt Use from Annual 1980–1986 Surveys*. Ottawa: Traffic Safety Standards and Research.

WAGENAAR, A. C., R. G. MAYBEE, and K. P. SULLIVAN. 1987. "Effects of Mandatory Seatbelt Laws on Traffic Fatalities in the United States." Ann Arbor: University of Michigan Transportation Research Institute.

WAGENAAR, A. C., L. J. MOLNAR, and K. L. BUSINSKI. 1987. "Direct Observation of Seat Belt Use in Michigan: July 1987." Ann Arbor: University of Michigan Transportation Research Institute.

WESTENBERG, DAVID. 1983. *Non-Use of Motor Vehicle Safety Belts as an Issue in Civil Litigation*. Washington, D.C.: National Highway Traffic Safety Administration.

WILLIAMS, A. F. 1982. "Passive and Active Measures for Controlling Heart Disease, Cancer, Stroke and Motor Vehicle Injuries: The Role of Health Psychologists." *Health Psychology* 1, no.4:399–409.

WILLIAMS, A. F., and B. O'NEILL. "Seat belt laws: Implications for Occupant Protection." SAE Technical Paper 2790683, Society of Automotive Engineers, Warrendale, Penn.

WILLIAMS, A. F., D. F. PREUSSER, R. D. BLOMBERG, and A. K. LUND, 1987a. "Results of a Seat Belt Use Law Enforcement and Publicity Campaign in Elmira, New York." *Accident Analysis & Prevention* 19, no. 4:243–49.

———. 1987b. "Seat Belt Use Law Enforcement and Publicity in Elmira, New York: A Reminder Campaign." *American Journal of Public Health* 77, no. 11:1450–51.

WILLIAMS, A. F., J. K. WELLS, and A. K. LUND. 1987. "Shoulder Belt Use in Four States with Belt Use Laws." *Accident Analysis & Prevention* 19, no.4:251–60.

WILLIAMS, A. F., J. K. WELLS, A. K. LUND, and N. TEED. 1987c. "Observed Use of Automatic Seat Belts in 1987 Cars." Washington, D.C.: Insurance Institute for Highway Safety.

WILLIAMS, J. B. 1987. "Safety Restraint Usage by Nebraska Drivers, Front Seat Passengers and Small Children Following Repeal of Required Usage Law." Lincoln: Nebraska Department of Motor Vehicles, Office of Highway Safety.

COMMENTS BY LEONARD EVANS

Individually, Chapter 2 by Campbell and Campbell and Chapter 3 by Williams and Lund provide the reader with an efficiently packaged and eminently readable compendium of information on consequences that flow from the passage of mandatory safety belt wearing laws in the United States. Together, they do the job even better, each complementing the other: Campbell and Campbell in Chapter 2 focus more on what has occurred, and Williams and Lund in Chapter 3 focus on what might occur in the future.

These authors document what might now be regarded as five firmly established effects:

1. Belt wearing rates increase after wearing is required by law.
2. Postlaw wearing rates settle to values higher than prelaw rates but lower than initial postlaw rates.
3. The magnitude of the increase in belt wearing rates is influenced by the degree of enforcement of the law; in particular, primary enforcement generates greater use rate increases than secondary enforcement.
4. Increases in use rates lead to observable reductions in the numbers of fatal and other injuries to vehicle occupants.
5. Fatality reductions tend to be less than calculated by simply scaling linearly the effectiveness of belts in crashes by the use rate increase.

These five effects are convincingly supported and documented in the papers, and I have essentially no substantial comments on the central themes of either paper. This being so, I could offer hearty congratulations to the authors and let the matter rest there. However, this would squander a forum generously provided by the organizers of the meeting, and would incidentally be somewhat out of character. Accordingly, I offer below some comments on more general themes, using at times the two subject papers for illustrative purposes.

The subject papers contain a few comments of an editorial nature. Rather than counter such comments where I would be inclined to do so, I prefer to offer some comments of my own, stressing that the opinions expressed are my own and not necessarily those of any other person, persons, let alone organizations. I hope that these comments might stimulate discussion on directions in which traffic safety research should aim. It is particularly appropriate to think about the future of the subject at a time when funding for new efforts has become available through the Centers for Disease Control. An immediate question is whether such funds should be spent in generating more activity of the same style and character as has occurred in the past, or whether we should be thinking along somewhat different lines. To answer such a question requires some perspective on the past.

In the more than 50 years since driving behavior and traffic safety were first analyzed in a technical way (Gibson and Crooks, 1938), much has been learned. However, when compared to advances in the traditional sciences in the same time span, increases in knowledge about traffic safety seem modest. The problem is not, as I see it, a lack of overall worldwide funding of what might be referred to in the most general terms as traffic safety research. Just about every jurisdiction in the motorized world appears to support some activity in data collection, codifying, examining, or analyzing that relates to traffic safety. Nor is it lack of quality or quantity of data; the observation of Gibson and Crooks (1938) that "accident statistics are now widely publicized" was already published in a journal more than half a century ago! Of course, in traffic safety research, as in any technical endeavor including the traditional sciences, one always desires more and better data. Below I discuss what I consider to be more intrinsic impediments to advancing understanding, in many cases building on published comments (Evans, 1985a; Hauer, 1987; Haight, 1985a, 1985b). In the interests of brevity and clarity, I indulge in much oversimplification, which I hope will not be mistaken for naivety.

Need for a Science of Traffic Safety

The most fruitful method to find out more about traffic safety is the same scientific method which has proven spectacularly successful in so many other fields. The primary motivation in science is curiosity, a desire to find out what is happening. All too often in traffic safety there appears to be insufficient recognition of the difference between knowledge, and what might be done with it. The scientific community should be dispassionately knowledgeable about, for example, the effect of alcohol on the probability that a driver will crash and on the probability that an intoxicated driver will be arrested (Ross, 1984). On the other hand, those pursuing the policy goal of trying to reduce harm from drunk driving may legitimately publicize the first of these items more than the second; it would be counterproductive to their goal to publicize that the probability of arrest for this offence is typically about one in two thousand, and that doubling police enforcement is consequently expected to increase the chances of arrest to one in one thousand.

Advocacy, by its very nature, implies making as good a case as you can. This involves selecting supporting evidence and leaving the task of presenting contrary evidence to opponents. Advocates generally consider evidence as something used to support previously held beliefs rather than providing the foundations of belief (Ross, 1987). Although advocacy may perform some functions well, it is nonetheless a process which is different from, and indeed inimical to, the normative processes in science. The goal aspired to in science is that all relevant evidence be evaluated in a detached and objective manner, and that the inquirer be "disinterested" in the result. The need for detached objectivity in evaluating countermeasures is particularly acute, and is persuasively argued by Ezra Hauer in his article "The Reign of Ignorance in Road Safety: A Case for Separating Evaluation from Implementation" (Hauer, 1987).

The question, What change in fatalities was associated with the passage of a mandatory belt law in some jurisdiction? is, in its structure, a simple factual question. Most would agree that there is an objective answer to this question embedded in nature. Although the answer may be difficult, or even impossible, to determine, it does not depend on the belief system, discipline, or training of the inquirer. This is not to suggest that science operates in a social vacuum; complex social factors determine what individuals, if any, are addressing this particular question, what methods they use, and what resources are available. However, such considerations do not invalidate my belief that the fatality change due to the law is not dependent to any important extent on the characteristics of those investigating it, and is, in principle, discoverable.

In contrast, the question, Ought we to pass (or enforce more strictly) mandatory belt wearing laws? is of a quite different nature and cannot be answered by science. Questions of this type are properly addressed through the workings of the political process, in which interests, beliefs, values, personal philosophies, and the right to legally pursue self-interest are legitimate ingredients. It is, however, expected that a more solid knowledge base will generally contribute to wiser policies.

I believe that the world is best served when the processes of science and advocacy are kept as separate as possible (Evans, 1988). Indeed, I see merit in going to some pains to delineate as clearly as possible whether one's proximate goal is the scientific one of finding out about nature, or the humanitarian one of doing good. Often pursuit of the scientific goal generates more good than the more frontal pursuit of good. Because of the historical intertwining of advocacy and research activities, those doing research must exercise particularly strong discipline to think and write as objectively as possible. It is a pity that the high research standards of the two subject papers should risk criticism for lack of objectivity of the type raised by Adams (1985a, p. 149) by occasional lapses into nonobjective language. For example, both subject papers liberally mention variables "improving," the term being applied to both fatality rates and belt-wearing rates. The reader is presumed to know that for fatality rates, improving means decreasing, whereas for belt-wearing rates it has the opposite meaning of increasing. In objective language, the values of measured quantities change; they can increase or they can decrease, but not improve. A problem possibly related to the above occurs in many tables in Campbell and Campbell (1988) which are, strictly speaking, incorrect; columns already labeled "fatality reductions" contain negative entries to indicate reductions.

The goals of a scientific examination of the effect of passing mandatory belt laws are first, to determine if there is any effect; second, to determine its sign; and third, to determine its magnitude. To use language which even hints that the first two questions might be answered by personal conviction alone adds credibility to the views of those who have a personal preference for the contrary belief that the laws have no effect on the total number of traffic deaths, or might even increase traffic fatalities (Adams, 1985a, 1985b).

Need to Create a Scientific Literature

All the traditional sciences accumulate knowledge in a clearly identifiable peer-reviewed, or refereed, literature. It is even more crucial that peer-reviewed literature be at the core of a subject such as traffic safety research, where so much is written for so many diverse purposes. Authors should feel reasonably comfortable (but not complacent) quoting results from such literature without the need to review all papers in detail; to require that all papers be read critically (which would involve similarly examining the work they cite, and so on) before citing would largely deny the field the possibility of advancing much beyond what one human mind can encompass. Work too recently performed to be already published in a peer-reviewed article makes a strong claim to be cited because of its currency; however, authors have a greater responsibility to examine unrefereed reports before using them, or even providing them the increased credibility of a citation. I believe we should strive for a goal in which any work more than a few years old that has not been accepted in a peer-reviewed journal should be ignored.

It should be stressed that I am here addressing papers which report research results. The comments do not apply to other areas, such as expressions of opinion, speculation, editorializing, etc. In particular, they do not apply to this article, which is clearly advocacy rather than science, or to many of the references cited in it.

Increasing the importance of peer-reviewed literature is the most effective way to discard the plethora of nonscientific "results" which overwhelm this field. The value of many papers is highly negative; not only do they spread misinformation but may oblige competent researchers to squander their time refuting nonsense. An additional benefit of peer review processes is that they militate against a clubiness in which some institutions attach more weight to the work of other institutions with which they have policy or financial entanglements.

What is crucially needed is an orderly expanding body of knowledge corresponding to the norm of traditional sciences. This is certainly not to say that work in peer-reviewed journals is of uniformly high quality, or even free from serious error; nor is it to deny that many important contributions have the *average* quality, importance, objectivity, and technical correctness of work appearing in such quality peer-reviewed journals as *Human Factors, Accident Analysis and Prevention, Journal of Safety Research and Risk Analysis,* compared to that in papers not subject to peer review. Given that there has been substantial literature in these very sources in the last few years, it is notable that 79 percent of the Campbell and Campbell (1988) references and 66 percent of the Williams and Lund (1988) references are to nonrefereed sources, many of them describing work now long superseded by findings in the refereed literature. I suspect the ease with which old reference lists can be pumped out on word processors contributed to this. As there is a need to reference legal statutes and the like, these percentages should not, even ideally, approach zero in traffic safety research. However, with the present state of knowledge, the percentages could have been lower.

Both subject papers discussed, in qualitative terms, differences between users and nonusers of safety belts. Not only have such effects been quantified (Evans, 1987a), but the result of this quantification has been used (Evans, 1987b) to derive the equation below which calculates fatality reductions expected from a change in safety belt use rates; to avoid confusion, this equation will hereafter be referred to as eqn 25, its number in Evans (1987b):

Percent reduction in fatalities

$$= \frac{20.2[u_f^3 - u_i^3 + 2.13\,(u_f - u_i)]}{1.47 - 0.43[u_i + 0.47u_i^3]} \qquad \text{eqn 25 of Evans (1987b)}$$

The only dependent variables which must be substituted into eqn 25 are the initial belt use rate, u_i, and the final belt use rate, u_f.

Table 3–A–1 shows a comparison of the predictions of eqn 25 with the observed fatality reductions as given in Figure 3–6 of Williams and Lund (1988), based on numerical values given in a reference they cite. Note that the observed fatality reductions are, for all four states, closer to the eqn 25 predictions than to predictions from the simple calculation, which assumes users and non-users have the same accident rates. Because I used a slightly different belt effectiveness value than Williams and Lund (1988), the simple calculation results in Table 3–A–1 differ slightly from their values. The effectiveness estimate I used (Evans, 1986) is more recent, is of higher precision, and was published in a peer-reviewed journal.

The reduction in the differences between observed values and those calculated using eqn 25 is the type of interplay between theory and observation which science is all about. A comparison of the observed fatality reductions with those calculated using eqn 25 generates no systematic difference such as displayed in Figure 3–6 of Williams and Lund (1988); three values are lower than predicted, and one is higher, with the average difference between predicted and observed being 1.5 percentage points. Eqn 25 does not capture all the effects which lead to actual fatality reductions differing from simple calculation predictions, but the closer agreement between theory and observation suggests a beginning understanding of what is going on. Eqn 25 also offers a quantitative explanation of part of the differences between other observed fatality changes, such as those in Campbell and Campbell (1988)

Table 3–A–1 Comparison of Calculated and Observed Fatality Reductions

State	Belt Use, %		Calculated Fatality Reduction, %[a]	Observed Fatality Reduction, %[b]	Fat. Reduction Estimated Using Simple Equation, %
	Before Law	After Law			
Illinois	18	42	8.4	5	11.2
New Jersey	17	42	8.7	6	11.6
Michigan	18	50	11.6	10	14.9
New York	12	52	14.1	16	18.1

[a]Calculated using eqn 25 of Evans (1987b).
[b]From Figure 3–6 of Williams and Lund (1988).

and Hedlund (1986), and those calculated using the simple equation.

Goal Is Quantification

A central goal in science is quantification. Regrettably, in traffic safety research (and all too many other subjects besides) this goal often appears to be replaced by the different, and often contradictory, goal of hypothesis testing. This can arise from inappropriate use or interpretation of statistical procedures. It seems to me that insufficient attention is paid to the following truisms: *For sufficiently small samples, no effect, no matter how large, is statistically significant. For sufficiently large samples, every effect, no matter how small or unimportant, becomes statistically significant.*

Expressing the results of a study in terms of the result of a hypothesis test may be more a commentary on the experiment than a statement about the effect under investigation. Quantitative estimates with error limits, say 20 ± 30 or 0.003 ± 0.001, convey crucial information immediately, whereas the statements, in isolation and devoid of quantitative estimate, that the first difference is not statistically significant whereas the second one is, while true, are rarely useful. Hypothesis testing has important applications, but mainly at the interface between total ignorance and the beginning of knowledge. Once we begin to know something about a phenomenon, we want to measure it quantitatively. To present data, such as the two examples below from Table 2–3 of Campbell and Campbell (1988), doesn't tell me what I really want to know:

State	Percent Change	Interv. signif.
Ill., Mich.	-6.0%	$p < .01$
Mass.	-9.4%	n.s.

At this stage of our knowledge, why should we focus so much attention on the probability that the true effect might be of sign opposite to the estimate? What I really want to know is the estimate, and its associated uncertainty (or in an alternate nomenclature, the point estimate and its associated confidence interval). To further illustrate the point, suppose we have four independent estimates of some quantity, perhaps from four unrelated studies, as follows: $(10 \pm 6)\%$, $(-1 \pm 8)\%$, $(7 \pm 5)\%$, and $(9 \pm 7)\%$, where the error is one standard error. Each of the four estimates falls well short, even at the low 0.1 level, of being statistically significantly different from zero. If all that was reported for each study was that the effect was not statistically significantly different from zero, then surely the naive reader must be forgiven for interpreting the consistent finding of no effect in each of four studies to constitute overwhelming evidence supporting no effect! That the reverse is so is readily apparent when one combines, using standard methods, the four quantitative values, and thereby obtains an overall composite estimate of $(7.0 \pm 3.1)\%$. When a quantitative estimate is available in this form, it is a simple matter to determine whether it is statistically significantly different from zero (or from any other value); the composite value is indeed statistically significantly different from zero ($p < 0.05$). Additional independent estimates can be similarly incorporated to yield a new composite estimate, so that the best estimate used at any time should be based on all prior estimates, and accordingly increase in precision as more studies are performed (see also, Hauer, 1983).

*   *   *

These comments have focused mainly on hopes that traffic safety research might in the future acquire more of the method, style, values, attitudes and institutional structures which have proved so successful in the traditional sciences, and that in the decades ahead understanding might increase at a greater rate than in the past. In advocating the application to traffic safety research of what might be called the normative model of science, I am not claiming that this model is in fact all that closely followed, even in the physical sciences. Even ignoring outright fraud, which Broad and Wade (1982) indicate is more common than generally recognized, the normative model of science is one which is subject to many criticisms (Kuhn, 1970; Feyerabend, 1975), being rarely the model used in the discovery process but more likely used to organize events after they have occurred. My claim is not so much that traditional science really follows this normative model, but that it is an understandable ideal standard. I believe that subjects which have such an idealized goal will make more progress than those which do not, because possession of such a standard enables more effective evaluation and criticism of contributions.

My plea that the normative, reductionist scientific method should become more central to traffic safety research is not to imply that other methods may never be used. There are many important areas devoid of data. I have previously offered the example of advising pedestrians to look both ways before crossing the road (Evans, 1985b), notwithstanding the absence of a shred of empirical justification for such a policy. Beyond questions of infeasible experiments, there may be other problems which are too complex and multifaceted to yield, at the present time at least, to the normative reductionist scientific method. Such problems include understanding why fatality rates have long-term downward trends in most countries (Evans, 1987d), why rates are different in different countries (Jacobs and Cutting, 1986; Adams, 1985b), and finding the relative contributions to youth crash overinvolvement of, on the one hand, inexperience and lack of skill, and on the other hand, characteristics intrinsic to youth (Evans, 1987c). I believe that at the moment the most fruitful approach to such problems involves a judgmental synthesis of available information, notwithstanding the potential pitfalls of relying on judgment in traffic safety matters which have been recently stressed by Hauer (1988). When we have little more than judgment and common sense to guide us, then I think they should be used, taking care to emphasize that this is the source. More solidly based specific information, which derives from the scientific method, contributes to advancing understanding in these broader areas. The process of synthesizing evolving information from many sources is more akin to the tradition of historical or social analyses than of normal science, and the conclusions derived are consequently vulnerable to criticism by those who disagree with them. What is to be avoided at all costs is the all too common practice of dressing opinions on traffic safety questions in indefensible, ad hoc, analyses to make them seem more solidly based than they are.

In closure, it seems appropriate to return to the two subject papers which provided the introduction for this piece. As promised, I have strayed much beyond these papers. In identifying many problems which have characterized the field, I have not meant to suggest, let alone imply, that these papers reflected them. I consider both these papers to contain a great deal of useful information. Each is a valuable addition to the literature on the subject, and I'm sure that I, and others, will be using them as valuable resources on many occasions in the future.

References

ADAMS, J. G. U. 1985a. *Risk and Freedom—The Record of Road Safety Regulations*. Nottingham, England: Transportation Publishing Projects, The Bottesford Press.

———. 1985b. "Smeed's Law, Set Belts and the Emperor's New Clothes." In L. Evans and R. C. Schwing (eds.), *Human Behavior and Traffic Safety*. New York: Plenum Press, pp. 193–248.

BROAD, W., and N. WADE. 1982. *Betrayers of the Truth*. New York: Simon and Schuster.

CAMPBELL, B. J., and F. A. CAMPBELL. 1988. "Injury Reduction and Belt Use Associated with Occupant Restraint Laws." Chapter 2 of this volume.

EVANS, L. 1985a. "Post Symposium Reflections" (comments on problems and issues in traffic safety research). In L. Evans and R. C. Schwing (eds.), *Human Behavior and Traffic Safety*. New York: Plenum Press, pp. 525–29.

———. 1985b. "Human Behavior Feedback and Traffic Safety." *Human Factors* 27:555–76.

———. 1986. "The Effectiveness of Safety Belts in Preventing Fatalities." *Accident Analysis and Prevention* 18:229–41.

———. 1987a. "Belted and Unbelted Driver Accident Involvement Rates Compared." *Journal of Safety Research* 18:57–64.

———. 1987b. "Estimating Fatality Reductions from Increased Safety Belt Use." *Risk Analysis* 7:49–57.

———. 1987c. "Young Driver Involvement in Severe Car Crashes." *Alcohol, Drugs and Driving* 3:63–78.

———. 1987d. "Factors Controlling Traffic Crashes." *The Journal of Applied Behavioral Science* 23: 201–18.

———. 1988. "The Science of Traffic Safety." *The Physics Teacher* (in press).

FEYERABEND, P. K. 1975. *Against Method: Outline of an Anarchistic Theory of Knowledge*. Atlantic Highlands, N.J.: Humanities Press.

GIBSON, J. J., and L. E. CROOKS. 1938. "A Theoretical Field-Analysis of Automobile Driving." *The American Journal of Psychology* 51:453–71.

HAIGHT, F. A. 1985a. "Road Safety: A Perspective and a New Strategy." *Journal of Safety Research* 16:91–98.

———. 1985b. "The Place of Safety Research in Transportation Research." *Transportation Research* 19A:373–76.

HAUER, E. 1983. "Reflections on Methods of Statistical Inference in Research on the Effect of Safety Countermeasures." *Accident Analysis and Prevention* 15: 275–85.

———. 1987. "The Reign of Ignorance in Road Safety: A Case for Separating Evaluation from Implementation." Paper presented to the Conference on Transportation Deregulation and Safety, Northwestern University, June 22–25, for publication in proceedings of the conference.

———. 1988. "A Case for Science-Based Safety Design and Management." Paper for presentation at ASCE specialty conference, Highway Safety at the Crossroads, March 28–30, San Antonio, Texas.

HEDLUND, J. 1986. "Casualty Reductions: Results from Safety Belt Use Laws." In *Effectiveness of Safety Belt Use Laws: A Multinational Examination*. U.S. Department of Transportation, National Highway Traffic Safety Administration, Report Number DOT HS 807 018, October.

JACOBS, G. D., and C. A. CUTTING. 1986. "Further Research on Accident Rates in Developing Countries." *Accident Analysis and Prevention* 18:119–27.

KUHN, T. S. 1970. *The Structure of Scientific Revolutions*. Chicago: University of Chicago Press.

ROSS, H. L. 1984. *Deterring the Drinking Driver*. Lexington, Mass. and Toronto: Lexington Books, D. C. Heath.

————1987. "Reflections on Doing Policy-Relevant Sociology: How to Cope with MADD Mothers." *The American Sociologist* 18:173–78.

WILLIAMS, A. F., and A. K. LUND. 1988. "Mandatory Seat Belt Use Laws and Occupant Crash Protection in the United States: Present Status and Future Prospects." Chapter 3 of this volume.

COMMENTS BY RALPH HINGSON

National reviews of the effects of seat belt legislation provided by Campbell and Williams clearly indicate that mandatory seat belt laws have reduced occupant injury and death. Between 1984 and early 1987, 32 states passed mandatory seat belt laws. However, two states, Massachusetts and Nebraska, have repealed such laws, and a binding referendum on Oregon's law is scheduled in 1988. That raises questions about whether seat belt laws might be repealed in other states.*

A close look at what happened in Massachusetts may provide insights into whether repeals are likely elsewhere. The Massachusetts law went into effect January 1, 1986 and applied to front and rear seat occupants, 5 years of age and older. As in two-thirds of states with laws, police were allowed to give citations only if the vehicle had been stopped for some other moving violation (secondary enforcement). The fine was $15. At least 10 states have fines of $15 or less.

Shortly after passage, opponents of the law secured a sufficient number of signatures to make the law subject to a binding referendum in November 1986, but a survey of 1,046 Massachusetts residents during the summer of 1986, while the law was in effect, revealed that 61 percent of respondents said they would vote to keep the law. Independent prelaw surveys yielded similar findings (Mass. Dept. of Public Health, 1985; Mass. Seat Belt Coalition, 1985). Nonetheless, the law was repealed in November by a 53 to 47 percent vote.

Repeal of the law within just two months of a statewide survey showing majority support for it raises the following important methodological and public policy questions:

- How strong was the support for the law during the summer of 1986?
- Were persons who favored the law in the summer of 1986 less likely to vote than those who opposed it?
- Did the 1986 survey miss people who voted against the law?
- Did voting respondents change their support for the law from the summer of 1986 to November, and if so, why?
- What effects did the law have on safety belt use and occupant injury and death?

---

*A more extensive analysis of the seat belt law repeal appears in *The American Journal of Public Health*, May 1988.

Methodological and Public Policy Questions

How Strong Was Support for the Law During the Summer of 1986?

Although 61 percent of 1,046 respondents in a statewide random digit dial telephone survey during the summer of 1986 (response rate of 72 percent) indicated they intended to vote to keep the law, only 42 percent said they strongly supported the law, and 61 percent said they believed the law invaded personal freedom. In the summer survey, respondents who did not always wear belts were asked whether a series of measures by the state would make them more likely to wear belts. The entire sample was also asked whether they supported or opposed those measures. Opposition was strongest for measures most likely, according to nonbelt-wearing respondents, to make them wear belts: stiffer fines, primary enforcement, and higher insurance costs for unbelted drivers. Support was greatest for education, the measure least likely, according to respondents, to stimulate use. In short, the public supported the law as passed with some concern about it invading personal liberty, but they were unwilling to adopt stiffer penalties or enforcement procedures to achieve high levels of compliance.

Did the Summer Survey Miss Opponents?

In December 1986, three weeks after the repeal, attempts were made to recontact all summer respondents to explore reasons for the repeal. Eighty percent interviewed during the summer were reinterviewed in December. That follow-up survey found that supporters and opponents were equally likely to vote, 62 versus 65 percent, respectively.

However, 64 percent of households that refused to be interviewed during the summer were also contacted after repeal, and 324 persons were interviewed. Fifty-eight percent said they voted on the repeal, 43 percent in favor and 47 percent against. In comparison, 53 percent of the voting summer respondents said they voted for keeping the law, and 45 percent voted for repeal. Thus, those summer survey refusers were less supportive of the law.

Did Voting Respondents Change Their Support?

Fifteen percent of voting summer supporters changed positions and voted to repeal the seat belt law, while only 4 percent of the summer opponents switched. The major reason for their change, cited by those who switched and voted for repeal, was that the law was an invasion of personal freedom. Perceptions that the law was not effective in reducing injury and death were also important. Questions concerning those issues were asked of respondents during the summer and after repeal. Persons who in December believed the law to be more of an invasion of personal liberty than they believed during the summer were seven times more likely than other respondents to switch from support to opposition. Also, those who in December saw the law as less effective than they had in the summer were five times more likely to switch and vote for repeal.

What Effects Did the Law Have on Belt Use and Occupant Injury and Death?

Repeat belt use observation surveys of over 10,000 motor vehicle occupants at 160 randomly selected signalized intersections state-wide revealed that when the seat belt law passed, belt use nearly doubled from 20 percent of occupants in December 1985 to 37 percent in February 1986, slipping slightly to 35 percent by August. This was considerably lower than reported postlaw use in many other belt law states. Moreover, according to the postlaw telephone survey, belt use was not adopted by respondents most likely to be drivers in crashes—namely, younger single males who drive more miles, drive more often after heavy drinking and drug use, and speed more often and run red lights. Eighty-seven percent who reported being in crashes during the time the law was in effect were not belted. As a result, motor vehicle occupant deaths declined only 4 percent per hundred million vehicle miles traveled during the eleven months the law was in effect compared to those same months the preceding year. In neighboring New England states without a belt law—Maine, New Hampshire, Vermont, and Rhode Island—belt use remained at 24 percent, and occupant deaths remained constant per 100 million vehicle miles traveled. Also, according to data from the Massachusetts Registry of Motor Vehicles, occupant serious and minor injuries declined 27 percent from 37,286 to 27,155 after the law, significantly greater than a 21 percent decline in nonoccupant injury. Though the postlaw Massachusetts occupant death declines were not statistically significant and were less than in other belt law states, they were consistent with some small beneficial effects of the law.

Discussion

The summer 1986 survey indicated greater support for the seat belt law than appeared in the November vote. The December 1986 survey indicated those persons who ultimately voted against the law were more likely to have refused to be interviewed in the summer survey. It is likely that biases introduced by survey refusal are not unique to Massachusetts but, rather, are relevant to all surveys on this issue.

However, an even more important reason for the unexpected repeal was that summer supporters were more likely than summer opponents to change their minds and vote for repeal. The postrepeal survey indicated the invasion of personal liberty and perceived ineffectiveness of the law are crucial issues on which a seat belt referendum can turn.

Regarding the effectiveness of belts within two weeks of the summer survey, the National Transportation Safety Board (1986) released a report on the potential dangers of rear seat lap belts. During the same week, the *Boston Globe* released a report that traffic deaths increased 10 percent after the Massachusetts law went into effect. People may tolerate some loss of personal liberty if they believe the sacrifice will achieve some benefit, but in the perceived absence of death reductions, seat belt laws may be viewed by many voters as requiring an unnecessary sacrifice of personal freedom.

To be sure, opposition to the law in Massachusetts was visible and resourceful. An Eastern Massachusetts radio talk show host, Jerry Williams, secured the 35,000 signatures needed to place the referendum on the November ballot. He debated proponents of the law on neutral forums and occasionally accepted their calls on his radio program. Although he indicated that he wore belts and encouraged others to do so, he maintained the law was an invasion of personal freedom. He predicted that primary enforcement, stiffer penalties for not wearing belts, and government intrusion into other areas like the workplace would follow if the belt law was not repealed. He contended that the law had been promoted by the automobile industry in an effort to avoid a federal requirement to install passive restraints in new vehicles and thus reduce costs. He argued that the law gave the police power to infringe on personal liberty and at one point erroneously broadcast that traffic jams on the Central Expressway, through Boston, were the result of police seat belt enforcement road blocks.

However, state efforts to maintain the law were also substantial. The Executive Office of Public Safety, the Governor's Highway

Safety Bureau, the Passenger Safety Program of the Massachusetts Department of Public Health, the Seat Belt Coalition, the Passenger Safety Association, the Registry of Motor Vehicles, and other professional organizations and service clubs participated in efforts to inform people of the law's components. One million information cards were printed and distributed statewide at turnpike booths and in schools. Highway signs were also posted. Almost immediately after the law went into effect, people who survived serious crashes because they wore belts were recruited to participate with the governor and local officials in public information campaigns. The Governor's Highway Safety Bureau assigned safety belt coordinators in five cities and recruited volunteers in 90 others across the state. Toll-free hot lines were set up to answer questions about belts. During the week prior to the election, advertisements supporting the law were aired statewide on network television. Over 25,000 citations for not wearing belts were issued by Massachusetts police.

That the law was repealed despite all these efforts suggests similar repeals can take place elsewhere. Massachusetts officials in many of their public statements and brochures about the law targeted a reduction of 100 deaths annually. That was clearly an overestimation. Even if Massachusetts had been able to achieve the 11 percent occupant death decline recently observed in Canadian provinces (Jonah and Lawson, 1984) or the 9 percent decline reported in New York (Williams and Lund, 1986), both of which have stiffer fines and primary enforcement, that would have resulted in sixty fewer deaths. One result of promising greater reductions in death and injury than could realistically have been achieved was that proponents were deprived of their strongest argument, the law's effectiveness. If in other states like Massachusetts, reductions in injury and death are less than promised, then even positive benefits may be viewed as disappointing.

The Massachusetts experience is similar in many respects to that of other states that enacted minimal penalties and secondary enforcement. Increases in belt use and decreases in injury and death have been substantially less than that observed in states with primary enforcement and more stringent penalties. If legislation in the United States is to have its full occupant protection potential, active law enforcement and meaningful penalties are essential.

States with secondary enforcement, minimal penalties, and low belt use levels are prime targets for repeal. In such states, death and injury reduction may lag far behind public expectations, just as they did in Massachusetts. That would deprive proponents of their strongest arguments to keep the laws. Even if the laws are not formally repealed, informal repeals measured by increased noncompliance with the laws could diminish their lifesaving benefits.

References

JONAH, B., and J. LAWSON. 1984. "The Effectiveness of Canadian Mandatory Seat Belt Laws." *Accident Analysis and Preview* 16:5.

Massachusetts Department of Public Health, Division of Family Health Services. 1985. *1984 Observational Survey Study*. Boston, Massachusetts Department of Public Health, March.

Massachusetts Seat Belt Coalition. 1985. "Surveys Indicate Massachusetts Drivers Favor Safety Belt Use Law by Two to One." News Release April 29, Boston.

National Transportation Safety Board. 1986. *Performance of Lap Belts in 26 Frontal Crashes*. Report No. NTSB/SS-86/03. Springfield, Va.: National Technical Information Service.

WILLIAMS, A. F., and A. K. LUND. 1986. "Seat Belt Use Laws and Occupant Crash Protection in the United States." *American Journal of Public Health* 76:1438–41.

Chapter 4

CHOOSING AUTOMATIC RESTRAINT DESIGNS FOR THE 1990s

by John D. Graham and Max Henrion

Introduction

In July 1984, the U.S. Department of Transportation (DOT) required all new cars sold in the United States to be equipped with automatic restraints by the 1990 model year. The rule also covers 10 percent of 1987 models, 25 percent of 1988 models, and 40 percent of 1989 models. If states comprising two-thirds of the population pass adequate mandatory belt use laws by April 1989, the rule will be automatically rescinded. Since few states have passed laws that are strong enough to pass DOT's criteria, it is likely that the rule will remain in effect into the 1990s (Williams and Lund, 1986).

The automatic restraint rule is a frontal crash performance standard that leaves compliance decisions in the hands of car producers. Based on recent production decisions and confidential interviews with industry officials, we believe that three automatic restraint designs are being seriously considered for the 1990s:

- Stationary, detachable, lap/shoulder belts, such as the design currently offered on the GM Buick Skylark (hereafter referred to as "detachable automatics");
- Motorized, nondetachable shoulder belts with knee pads (or manual lap belts) such as the designs currently offered on the

Toyota Cressida and Ford Escort (hereafter referred to as "motorized automatics"); and
- Combination driver-passenger air bag systems ("twin air bags") in conjunction with manual lap/shoulder belts.

DOT has encouraged car producers to develop the air bag technology by allowing a driver-side air bag (accompanied by manual lap/shoulder belts on the driver and passenger sides) to satisfy the rule through model year 1989 (NHTSA, 1987).

In this chapter we simulate the lifesaving and economic consequences of alternative design choices for model year 1990 cars. Our analysis is intended to provide information relevant to the following questions:

- Are automatic restraints desirable in a mixed environment of voluntary and mandatory belt use and, if so, which design is preferable?
- What research should be conducted in the next several years to assist decision makers in both DOT and the auto industry as they consider automatic-restraint policy for the 1990s?

We begin with the selection of two value frameworks, proceed with a description of two corresponding simulation models, continue with a presentation of modeling results and key sources of uncertainty, and conclude with a discussion of research and regulatory implications.

Value Frameworks

Since regulatory and research policy cannot be made in a value-neutral fashion, we have selected two value frameworks as a basis for the simulation models that follow. The *lifesaving framework* assumes that society wants to choose the automatic restraint design that will maximize the number of lives saved. In contrast, the *economic framework* assumes that society wants to choose the automatic restraint design that will maximize the difference between economic benefits and costs. Both value frameworks have a plausible basis, and together they capture much of the range in value positions that dominate controversies about health and safety regulation.

Simulation Models

In this section we describe simulation models designed to quantify the lifesaving and economic consequences of alternative restraint designs. The models, which are modified versions of our earlier work published in *Risk Analysis* (Graham and Henrion, 1984), are distinguished by the formal quantification of uncertainty about model inputs and outputs. Uncertainty is expressed in subjective probabilistic form in accordance with the tenets of Bayesian decision theory (Raiffa, 1968).

Lifesaving Model

Our first model expresses lives saved (L) as a function of a projected base case fatality rate for 1990 cars (b); an effectiveness rate for each restraint system in fatality prevention (E_f); a usage rate for each system in crashes (U) under three legal environments—strong (S) law, weak (W) law, and no (N) law; and a projection of the fraction (F) of a vehicle's life subject to alternative legal environments (where $F_S + F_W + F_N = 1.0$). For each restraint system, we estimate the number of lives saved over the car's life as

$$L = bE_f U$$

where $\qquad\qquad U = U_S F_S + U_W F_W + U_N F_N$

Economic Model

Our second model is slightly more complicated because it incorporates information about both the costs and benefits of alternative restraint designs. The net benefits of each restraint system are modeled as a function of lives saved (L); nonfatal injuries prevented (I); the economic value of saving a statistical life (V); the equivalence ratio for fatalities and nonfatal injuries (R); the unit capital and operating costs (C) of each restraint system, and projected 1990 car sales (S). For each system we estimate net benefits as

$$NB = (L + I/R) V - CS$$

where L, I, and C are expressed as present value figures using an uncertain real discount rate (D). The base case fatalities and operating costs are distributed over a 15-year vehicle life using R. L. Polk Company's car survival data before present values are computed (MVMA, 1985).

Values of Input Variables

We have assigned each input variable a subjective probability (or "credibility") distribution based on our earlier work, our interpretation of NHTSA's *Regulatory Impact Analysis* (NHTSA, 1984), and our knowledge of the relevant literature. Table 4–1 summarizes the values of key input variables that we have used. We invite comment on whether these numbers are plausible and whether the credibility ranges are too wide or too narrow. The range covered by the 0.1 and 0.9 fractiles corresponds to an 80 percent credibility interval. The 0.50 fractile corresponds to the median of our subjective credibility distribution.

Simulation Technique

The probability distributions obtained for the input variables induce probability distributions over the two outcome variables: lives saved and net benefits. The outcome distributions were computed by the Demos modeling system using Monte Carlo simulation with 200 points.

The probability distributions for those input variables constrained to be in the unit interval, 0 to 1.0, are modeled as log-odds-normal distributions. For quantity X, the distribution of log $(X/1-X)$ is assumed normal. This distribution has properties similar to the beta distribution: symmetric for quantities with median 0.5 and skewed toward the middle for quantities with median much smaller or larger than 0.5. Combinations of such variables are also performed in the log-odds form, when the standard manipulations on normal distributions can be carried out.

In generating probability distributions for input variables, we have assumed various probabilistic dependencies. For each restraint system, E_I is assumed to be slightly larger than E_f, but the two quantities are strongly correlated. We first generated E_f and then E_I by adding a small uncertain quantity with a median of five percentage points, representing the difference in the two quantities. Since E_I is generated from E_f, their dependence is large.

Similarly, the E's for all systems are highly correlated because they are assumed to be dependent on common biomechanical factors. We first generated E_f for lap/shoulder belts and then reduced it by an uncertain quantity with median 2.5 percentage points to generate E for motorized shoulder belts/knee pads. We reduced it by a larger quantity to obtain E for air bags alone, and increased it slightly for the combination of air bags and lap/shoulder belts.

Usage rates for each restraint system are also generated so as to be positively correlated. U for manual belts with strong laws is the base, from which U's for the automatic systems are derived. U in a

Table 4–1   Values of Input Variables

Input Variables	Fractiles of Credibility Distribution		
	0.10	0.50	0.90
E_f = Fatality effectiveness (%)			
lap shoulder belt	40	45	50
shoulder belt/knee pads	33	43	50
air bag only	20	28	41
air bag & lap/shoulder belt	44	50	56
E_I = Injury effectiveness (%)			
lap/shoulder belt	45	50	55
shoulder belt/knee pads	39	48	56
air bag only	23	33	46
air bag & lap/shoulder belt	48	55	61
U = Restraint use (%)			
manual lap/shoulder belt			
Voluntary	5	9	16
Weak law	21	29	41
Strong law	40	50	60
nondetachable motorized shoulder belt			
Voluntary	72	86	94
Weak law	76	87	95
Strong law	82	89	95
detachable automatic lap/shoulder belt			
Voluntary	10	17	30
Weak law	25	34	45
Strong law	45	55	65
belt use in cars with air bags as a percentage of manual lap/shoulder belt use (%)	60	84	95
air bag readiness factor (%)	98	98	98
F = Fraction of cars in states with belt use legislation (%)			
Voluntary	5	19	50
Weak law	22	38	54
Strong law	19	40	55
Weak or strong law	50	81	95
V, R = Economic value of injury Prevention			
Fatality ($M/life)	0.5	1.6	5.0
Injury-to-fatality equivalence ratio	25	50	100
C = Present value of economic costs (capital and operating) of restraint systems ($)			
Manual lap/shoulder belts	60	73	90
Motorized shoulder belt/knee pads	180	200	225
Stationary, detachable automatic lap/shoulder belt	90	104	120
Twin air bag systems (driver & passenger)	300	417	580
D = Real discount rate (%)	1	5	9
b = Base case death rate (deaths/10,000 registered cars)	16.5	19.3	23.4
S = 1990 car sales (10_6)	8.0	10.0	12.0

strong law environment is reduced by progressively larger decrements to obtain *U*'s for weak-law and no-law environments. The actual distributions for the uncertain decrements vary for the three automatic restraint systems, but the decrements are totally correlated. If a change in legislation affects usage rates for one system, we assume it will do so for the other systems as well.

Uncertainties about the distributions of cars in states with various legal environments were also assumed to be dependent. The fraction of cars under voluntary laws was generated as a log-odds normal with 80 percent credible interval from 5 to 50 percent; then the remaining fraction was divided into strong and weak law groups using a second uncertain fraction (a log-odds normal with 80 percent credible interval from 35 to 63 percent). In this way, the three fractions are guaranteed to sum to one.

Results

The estimated lifesaving consequences of alternative design choices are reported in Table 4–2. These estimates are calculated with reference to manual belts in a mixed voluntary-compulsory usage environment. Given our modeling assumptions, motorized automatics are estimated to save the most lives, followed by air bags and then detachable automatics.

The estimated economic consequences of alternative design choices are reported in Table 4–3. Again, calculations are made relative to manual belts. The same ranking of designs occurs at the median of the estimates. However, air bags are estimated to pose a chance (about 0.20) of negative net benefits.

A more direct method of comparison is to compute the difference in lives saved and net benefits for pairs of restraint systems.

Table 4–2   Lifesaving Consequences of Alternative Automatic Restraint Programs

Type of Automatic Restraint	Estimated Lives Saved in 1990 Model Cars* Fractiles of Credibility Distribution		
	0.10	0.50	0.90
Detachable, automatic lap/shoulder belt	360	505	840
Nondetachable, motorized shoulder belt/ knee pads	2,800	4,200	590
Full-front air bags with manual lap/ shoulder belts	2,400	3,600	5,500

*Estimates made relative to manual lap/shoulder belts.

Table 4–3   Economic Consequences of Alternative Automatic Restraint
Programs

Type of Automatic Restraint	Estimated Present Value of Net Benefits* (in billions of 1984 dollars) Fractiles of Credibility Distribution		
	0.10	0.50	0.90
Detachable, automatic lap/ shoulder belt	$0.04 B.	$0.86 B.	$3.30 B.
Nondetachable, motorized shoulder belt/knee pads	$1.40	$8.30	$27.40
Full-front air bags with manual lap/shoulder belts	$ − 1.10	$4.60	$23.60

*Calculated relative to manual belt designs.

Table 4–4   Estimated Difference in Lives Saved and Net Benefits for
Alternative Restraint Designs

Restraint Comparison	Outcome Variable	Fractiles of Credibility Distribution		
		0.10	0.50	0.90
Motorized Automatics:	L	2328	3621	5014
Detachable Automatics	NB	$ 1.09 B.	$ 6.09 B.	$23.6 B.
Twin Air Bags:	L	− 2290	−660	1380
Motorized Automatics	NB	$ − 10.00 B.	$ − 3.4 B.	$ 1.2 B.
Twin Air Bags:	L	1760	3080	5000
Detachable Automatics	NB	$ − 1.50 B.	$ 3.30 B.	$19.7 B.

Results from that exercise are reported in Table 4–4. The results
confirm the finding that motorized automatics are more promising
than both detachable automatics and air bags under each value
framework.

Key Sources of Uncertainty

In order to chart research priorities, it would be useful to know
which uncertain input variables contribute the most to uncertainty
about lives saved and net benefits. Those uncertain variables that
do not contribute significantly to uncertainty about outputs may
deserve low priority in policy-related research. Alternatively, the
input variables responsible for the greatest amount of uncertainty
about lives saved and net benefits may deserve high priority in
research policy.

In order to identify key sources of uncertainty, we computed
the Spearman's rank correlation of the sample values for output

quantities (lives saved and net benefits) with those of each of the uncertain input quantities (*U, E, F, V* and so forth). The rank order correlation differs from ordinary correlation only in that we are looking at the correlation of the ranks of the values for each quantity rather than the values themselves. The advantage of the rank-based correlation is that it is not unduly affected by extreme outliers on the tails of input and output distributions.

The rank correlations are a measure of the direction and relative size of the contribution of each uncertain input to the output. They provide a method for comparing the relative importance of the different uncertain inputs. In many policy analysis models only a few uncertain inputs contribute most of the uncertainty while the rest contribute negligibly.

The results of our correlation analysis are presented in Table 4–5, where the reported correlation coefficients are based on 200 sample points. In the case of the lifesaving model, the uncertainty about the difference in lives saved by restraint designs is determined primarily by uncertainty about effectiveness rates for automatic restraints. Usage rates are a less important source of uncertainty. For the economic model, the economic value of lifesaving (*V*) emerges as a crucial source of uncertainty. *E* is again a significant source of uncertainty. *C* for air bags and motorized belts is also a significant source of uncertainty.

Policy and Research Implications

During the next several years, car producers and the National Highway Traffic Safety Administration (NHTSA) will make some crucial decisions about the future of automatic restraints. Our analysis, rough as it is, raises some significant findings and questions relevant to such decisions.

First, all three automatic restraint designs appear to be more promising than manual belt designs, even in a legal environment where many states compel belt use. This finding persists under both value frameworks.

Second, the three automatic restraint designs are not equally promising. In particular, detachable automatics appear to offer less lifesaving and fewer net benefits than motorized automatics. We recommend that car producers and NHTSA take a careful look at whether current policies are too permissive toward detachable automatics. If consumer resistance to motorized systems is anticipated (despite their apparent popularity), it would seem that air

Table 4–5   Input Variables That Contribute Significantly to Uncertainty About Lives Saved and Net Benefits

Restraint Comparison	Input Variables with Significant Spearman's Rank Correlation Coefficient	Absolute Size of Coefficient
I. *Lifesaving Model*		
Motorized Automatics: Detachable Automatics	1. E_f (motorized automatics)— E_f (detachable automatics)	0.65
	2. U (motorized automatics)— U (detachable automatics)	0.45
Twin Air Bags: Motorized	1. E_f (air bags alone)— E_f (motorized automatics)	0.73
	2. E_f (lap/shoulder belt)— E_f (motorized automatic)	0.45
	3. U (motorized automatics)— U (lap/shoulder belt)	0.36
Twin Air Bags: Detachable Automatics	1. E_f (air bags)— E_f (detachable automatics)	0.78
	2. E_f (lap/shoulder belt)	0.42
	3. U (lap/shoulder belts/air bag)— U (lap/shoulder belt)	0.26
II. *Economic Model*		
Motorized Automatics: Detachable Automatics	1. V (economic value of saving a statistical life)	0.92
Twin Air Bags: Motorized Automatics	1. E_f (air bags alone)— E_f (motorized automatics)	0.63
	2. V (economic value of saving a statistical life)	0.18
	3. C (air bags)	0.28
	4. C (motorized automatics)	0.36
Twin Air Bags: Detachable Automatics	1. V (economic value of saving a statistical life)	0.84
	2. E (air bags)— E (detachable automatics)	0.31
	3. C (twin air bags)	0.26
	4. C (motorized automatics)	0.26

bag systems would be a better alternative than detachable automatics.

Third, our analysis does not produce a definitive finding on the relative merits of motorized automatics and air bags, although motorized systems appear to have an edge in both models. To clarify this situation, we recommend that NHTSA and car producers undertake careful analysis of the relative effectiveness and costs of motorized automatics (both those that include knee pads and those that incorporate manual lap belts), and air bags. Additionally, we urge NHTSA and car producers to monitor carefully the rate of manual belt use in cars with air bags in order to detect slippage and target educational efforts.

Finally, NHTSA should consider whether it would be desirable in the long run to write two standards—one requiring (motorized?) automatic belts and the other requiring air bags. In particular, we believe it would be unfortunate if the momentum building in favor of air bags would cause the demise of motorized automatics in the 1990s.

In order to consider seriously air bags as a supplement to motorized belts, answers to at least the following questions are necessary:

- How much extra safety (fatal and nonfatal risk reduction) does the air bag offer to restrained occupants?
- How much is air bag crash performance hindered by the absence of a lap belt (either because it isn't used or is replaced by knee pads)?

Precise answers to these questions must await the large-scale field test of air bags that is now being launched.

References

GRAHAM, J. D., M. HENRION. 1984. "A Probabilistic Analysis of the Passive-Restraint Question." *Risk Analysis* 4:25–40.

Motor Vehicle Manufacturer Association (MVMA). 1985. *Facts and Figures 1984*. Detroit: MVMA.

National Highway Traffic Safety Administration (NHTSA). 1984. *Final Regulatory Impact Analysis: Amendment to Federal Motor Vehicle Safety Standard Number 208 Passenger Car Front Seat Occupant Protection*. Washington, D.C.: U.S. Dept. of Transportation.

———. 1987. "Denial of Petition for Reconsideration." *Federal Registrar* 52:42440.

RAIFFA, HOWARD. 1970. *Decision Analysis: Introductory Lectures on Choices under Uncertainty*. Reading, Mass.: Addison-Wesley.

WILLIAMS, A. F., and A. K. LUND. 1986. "Seat Belt Use and Occupant Crash Protection in the United States." *American Journal of Public Health* 76:1438–42.

COMMENTS BY BARRY FELRICE

Graham and Henrion have done an admirable job in identifying those factors that enable decision makers to judge the relative merits of alternatives. For automatic occupant protection devices, the input variables of device effectiveness when used, usage (or readiness, as is the case for air bags), and the effect of different types of state belt laws, completely define the benefit side of any type of benefit-cost analysis. Similarly, the lifetime costs of the several devices (purchase price plus operating costs) and the values associated with avoiding injuries or deaths complete the cost side. Finally, the two simulation models of lifesaving and economics comprise the totality of ways of examining the issue—that is, does one attempt to maximize benefits (deaths and injuries avoided) or to optimize in terms of net costs (after placing a dollar value on deaths and injuries)? The authors have done a thorough job in identifying the input variables to their models, portraying the outputs in a concise fashion, and examining the results in terms of sensitivities to some of the input variables. This sensitivity analysis is a strong point of their work.

In reviewing Graham's and Henrion's work, I first noted that all the possible permutations of automatic restaint devices were not included in the analysis. The paper compares air bags to manual lap/shoulder belts, to nondetachable motorized belts, and to detachable lap/shoulder automatic belts. However, automatic belts come in many shapes and forms. They may be two-point (shoulder belt only) or three-point (lap and shoulder belt). They may be motorized or nonmotorized. And, they may be detachable or nondetachable. Thus, a matrix of six types of automatic belts is possible. Indeed, four types are already on the market—the two analyzed in the paper plus stationary, detachable shoulder-only belts (Hyundai Excel, VW Golf/Jetta, and Yugo GVL and GVX) and motorized detachable shoulder belts (Nissan Maxima).

I believe that expanding the analysis to include these other systems would enhance the value of Graham and Henrion's work. For example, is it the motorized aspect of certain belts which results in high usage, the nondetachability aspect, or some combination of the two? The Nissan detachable motorized belt appears to have similar usage to the Toyota nondetachable motorized system, indicating that the detachability aspect may be unimportant, at least for motorized systems. Stationary detachable system usage varies from the three-point GM system (65 percent) to Chrysler's two-point system (45 percent) to VW's two-point system with interlock (90 percent). Obviously, factors other than whether the belt is detachable or even two- versus three-point are at play.

101

While all six permutations are not offered for sale, an examination of the four that are would aid in a more complete evaluation.

As a further analysis, it would be useful to analyze the consequences of driver-side air bags and passenger manual belts. While not a permanent option under the standard, it is permitted until September 1, 1993, not just through the 1989 model year (September 1, 1989) as Graham and Henrion state.

As with any modeling effort, the outputs are only as good as the inputs. While most of the values for the inputs are certainly within expected ranges, others deserve additional clarification or explanation. For example, the usage rates of both manual and automatic belts are shown to be dependent on whether a state has a strong, weak, or no mandatory belt usage law. Yet the authors never define what criteria were used to classify states according to this system. Restraint usage for manual lap/shoulder belts in states without a usage law ranges from 5 to 16 percent in the analysis. However, the most recent NHTSA survey shows average driver belt usage in no-law states to be 27 percent. While usage in crashes may be lower than average observed usage, the range used in the model appears to be rather narrow.

Similarly, the analyzed range of usage in seat belt law states appears small. Best estimate usage values of 29 to 50 percent are shown for weak and strong law states, respectively. However, average usage values of greater than 50 percent and, in some states higher than 70 percent, have recently been observed. Some explanation of why these current values are deemed outside even the 90 percent fractile would enable the reader to better assess the figures used in the analysis.

The detachable automatic belt figures also appear low. As stated earlier, Nissan's motorized automatic detachable belt has been observed with over 80 percent usage. Recent surveys by the Insurance Institute for Highway Safety and NHTSA have shown usage of the GM three-point detachable system to be from 40 to nearly 80 percent. Yet, in the analysis, only in states with the undefined "strong" laws is usage shown to ever exceed 45 percent.

I would also question why the authors believe belt use in cars with air bags is expected to be 16 percent lower than in cars without them. While the "air bag as panacea" theory could account for this, the safety consciousness of people who voluntarily purchase air bag cars could actually lead to *higher* usage than exists in nonair bag cars.

The cost figures appear not to raise many questions except that the costs of motorized belt systems as reported by manufacturers are much higher than the $127 shown in the analysis. Differential costs of motorized versus manual belt systems are $200 to $300, as reported by the auto companies. Conversely, the full front air bag expected cost of $417 is quite a bit higher than NHTSA's estimate of $330 and even lower estimates quoted recently by suppliers. The latter two items seem to bias unfairly the analysis against air bags and for motorized belt systems.

Graham and Henrion conclude that NHTSA (among others) will be making crucial decisions in the next few years regarding automatic restraints and recommends that NHTSA consider requiring motorized automatic belts and air bags. While economic theory seeks to *maximize* net benefits, safety regulations do not. Instead, regulations seek to protect the public against "unreasonable risk" of harm through the setting of *minimum performance* standards. The minimum nature of such standards argues that the government is not soon likely to reopen rule making on this subject.

Even more important is the prohibition in the statute and its legislative history regarding the setting of "design" standards. The Senate report stated:

> *Unlike the General Service Administration's procurement standards, which are primarily design specifications, [safety] standards are expected to be performance standards, specifying the required minimum safe performance of vehicles but not the manner in which the manufacturer is to achieve the specified performance. Manufacturers and parts suppliers will thus be free to compete in developing and selecting devices and structures that can meet or surpass the performance standard.*
>
> *Such safety performance standards are thus not intended or likely to stifle innovation in automotive design.*

The Conference Committee report reiterated this theme more succinctly: "The Secretary is not to become directly involved in questions of design."

The performance nature of the automatic occupant protection standard has led to the myriad designs now in the marketplace. To take a slice in time and presume that one device is superior over another misses the point that some means of compliance, which may be superior to all that now exist, is yet to be developed. Indeed, the motorized belt system which the authors find superior would not have even been permitted had the original requirement for air cushion restraints not been changed to the more performance-oriented automatic restraint standard.

Thus, while Graham and Henrion appear to regret that the rule "leaves compliance decisions in the hands of car producers," the law requires this. Furthermore, the various designs used by different manufacturers not only make a study such as this feasible—and the analysis method contained therein should prove useful to manufacturers, insurers, etc.—but correctly leads to increased safety competition. Again, given the contentious nature of the 20-year battle for automatic restraints—and the reality of their finally appearing in large numbers of cars—NHTSA is very unlikely to consider any near-term changes to its regulation.

COMMENTS BY BRIAN O'NEILL

Graham and Henrion address several questions related to the lifesaving and economic consequences of alternative automatic restraint design choices. Two value frameworks—life saving and economic—were selected, and simulation models for each were developed. The results from the modeling were then used to discuss the policy and research implications. The literature contains few examples of attempts to develop the policy implications of alternative occupant restraint design choices using an analytic framework, and Graham and Henrion deserve some praise for trying to address this issue.

Although the models themselves may be adequate, the values used for several of the key input variables are at best educated guesses. In particular, the effectiveness of two-point motorized belts with knee bolsters and the costs of the different restraint systems are simply not known with any certainty; yet the conclusions of the paper depend completely on the values assumed for these parameters. The two models are inappropriately complicated, given that values for many of the input parameters do not exist. Better insight into the questions raised by Graham and Henrion can be obtained by much simpler and straightforward analyses.

It is important to recognize that several basic designs for automatic seat belts have been used by the various car manufacturers to date (Table 4–A–1). The motorized designs—both detachable and nondetachable—all include knee bolsters and manual lap belts. The nonmotorized designs vary somewhat more and include detachable lap/shoulder belts; detachable shoulder belts with knee bolsters and manual lap belts; and detachable shoulder belts with ignition interlocks, knee bolsters, and no lap belts.

Williams et al. (1987) observed seat belt use in four metropolitan areas for new cars with various automatic systems and corresponding models with manual belts (Table 4–A–2). In every case, except for the Chrysler automatic belt system, shoulder belt use was higher in the cars with automatic belts than in the corresponding models with manual belts. The motorized two-point automatic belts and the VW system had use levels of about 90 percent; the GM detachable lap/shoulder belt system had 64 percent usage. Table 4–A–3 shows lap belt use in the cars with automatic belts. The GM system produced the highest overall rate of lap/shoulder belt use (65 percent); in the cars with manual lap belts, use ranges from about 30 to nearly 50 percent.

These results indicate that shoulder belt use is highest in the cars with two-point systems that are either motorized or have ignition interlocks, but manual lap belt use in these cars—when a lap belt is available—is considerably lower. This difference raises

Table 4–A–1 Automatic Belt System in 1987 Cars

Type	Use Characteristics	Manufacturer (Models)
I. *Motorized shoulder belt*		
Nondetachable shoulder belt with manual lap belt and knee bolster	Shoulder belt moves along guide rail in roof of car and positions itself around occupant when door is closed and ignition turned on; minimal or no contact with occupant entering or exiting car; can be disabled permanently by cutting or unbolting; shoulder belt cannot be used as a manual belt.	Ford Motor Company (Escort, Mercury Lynx) Toyota Motor Sales, U.S.A., Inc. (Camry, Cressida)
Detachable shoulder belt with manual lap belt and knee bolster	Shoulder belt moves along guide rail in roof of car and positions itself around occupant when door is closed and ignition turned on; minimal or no contact with occupant when entering and exiting car; can be detached from the guide rail and used as a manual belt.	Nissan Motor Corporation, U.S.A. (Maxima)
II. *Nonmotorized shoulder belt*		
Detachable shoulder belt with manual lap belt and knee bolster	Shoulder belt attached to door and wraps around occupant when door is closed; some contact with occupant when entering or exiting car; can be detached where the belt attaches to the door and used as a manual belt.	Chrysler Corporation (LeBaron Coupe, Dodge Daytona)
Detachable shoulder belt with knee bolster but no lap belt	Shoulder belt attached to door and wraps around occupant when door is closed; some contact with occupant when entering and exiting car; must be attached to start car but can be detached after car is started.	Volkswagen United States, Inc. (Golf, Jetta)
III. *Nonmotorized lap and shoulder belt*	Three-point lap/shoulder belt system attached to door and wraps around occupant when door is closed; some contact with both lap and shoulder portions when entering and exiting car; can be disconnected via inboard buckle and used as a manual lap/shoulder belt.	General Motors Corporation (Buick LaSabre, Skylark, Somerset; Oldsmobile Calais, Delta 88; Pontiac Bonneville, Grand Am)

Table 4–A–2 Percent of Front Seat Occupants Using Shoulder Belts in Late Model Cars Equipped with Manual or Automatic Belt Systems

Manufacturer and Belt Type	Washington, D.C.		Chicago		Los Angeles		Philadelphia		All Areas	
	%	N	%	N	%	N	%	N	%	N
Chrysler										
Manual	72	(64)	68	(50)	77	(44)	39	(107)	59	(265)
Automatic	67	(9)	53	(19)	50	(22)	32	(31)	46	(81)
Ford										
Manual	67	(302)	49	(539)	59	(164)	39	(343)	52	(1,348)
Automatic	92	(86)	84	(240)	87	(76)	88	(138)	87	(540)
GM										
Manual	66	(600)	55	(1,380)	63	(387)	41	(815)	55	(3,182)
Automatic	76	(99)	64	(554)	77	(115)	47	(180)	64	(948)
Nissan										
Manual	71	(173)	57	(165)	67	(216)	52	(143)	63	(697)
Automatic	93	(70)	91	(101)	88	(138)	81	(79)	88	(388)
Toyota										
Manual	79	(170)	73	(180)	73	(181)	66	(96)	74	(627)
Automatic	97	(220)	96	(353)	95	(417)	98	(167)	96	(1,157)
VW										
Manual	72	(249)	63	(200)	63	(311)	60	(236)	64	(996)
Automatic	86	(49)	95	(21)	92	(26)	87	(38)	89	(134)

Table 4–A–3 Percent of Drivers Using Lap Belts in Late Model Cars Equipped with Automatic Belt Systems

Manufacturer and Lap Belt Type	Washington		Chicago		Los Angeles		Philadelphia		All Areas	
	%	N	%	N	%	N	%	N	%	N
Chrysler Manual	56	(9)	39	(18)	35	(20)	16	(25)	32	(72)
Ford Manual	48	(75)	29	(201)	39	(64)	38	(115)	36	(455)
GM Automatic	75	(84)	65	(476)	79	(98)	49	(155)	65	(813)
Nissan Manual	50	(62)	36	(84)	51	(110)	27	(64)	42	(320)
Toyota Manual	53	(180)	42	(306)	54	(331)	41	(132)	48	(949)

the question of how to compare the lifesaving benefits from high automatic shoulder belt use and lower manual lap belt use with lap/shoulder belt use that is higher than the manual lap belt use but lower than the automatic shoulder belt use, as is the case with the GM system. The fatality-reducing effectiveness of lap/shoulder belts has been well established and is generally accepted to be about 45 percent. Using this estimate, the expected percentage reductions in fatalities for different levels of belt use in crashes*

---

*Belt use in crashes is typically lower than belt use observed in the general driving population.

increases linearly from 0 with no belt use to 45 percent at 100 percent belt use (Figure 4–A–1). Two-point belts with knee bolsters are thought to be less effective than three-point belts, but precisely how much less effective has not been established. In the final supporting materials for automatic restraint regulations, the U.S. Department of Transportation (DOT) suggested a *lower bound* for the effectiveness of two-point belts of 35 percent (U.S. NHTSA, 1984). That estimate is used in Figure 4–A–1 to illustrate the relationship between belt use and fatality reductions for two-point systems with *no* manual lap belt use.

As shown in Figure 4–A–1, a 31 percent reduction in fatalities can be expected from 90 percent use of two-point automatic belts, which is the use rate observed in such cars when new. For three-point belts to achieve a comparable fatality reduction, use would have to be 70 percent; if usage of three-point belts is lower, two-point belts produce greater fatality reductions; if three-point belt use is higher, they achieve greater fatality reductions. It is important to remember, however, that these comparisons assume that there is no manual lap belt use in the cars with two-point automatic belts, and we know that this is not the case in practice.

As manual lap belt use increases from 0 to 90 percent, the expected fatality reduction with 90 percent use of two-point auto-

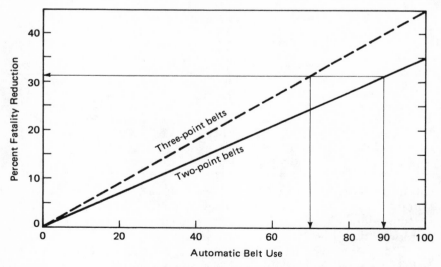

Figure 4-A-1   Comparative Reductions in Fatalities for Three-Point Automatic Belts and Two-Point Automatic Belts with No Lap Belt Use. Based on midpoint of effectiveness range (40-50 percent) estimated for three-point belts and lowest effectiveness (35 percent) estimated for two-point belts.

matic belts increases from 31 percent to just over 40 percent, or the same reduction that would be expected from 90 percent use of lap/shoulder belts. In Williams et al. (1987), manual lap belt use in cars with two-point belts ranged from about 25 to 55 percent in the four metropolitan areas. As shown in Figure 4–A–2, lap belt use at these levels increases the expected fatality reduction with automatic two-point belts to 34 or 37 percent, depending on lap belt usage. To achieve equivalent fatality reductions, use of three-point automatic belts would have to be 75 or 82 percent. The lower of these two levels was barely achieved in two of the four metropolitan areas surveyed; overall use was 64 percent.

Thus, the automatic shoulder belts should produce greater fatality reductions than the automatic lap/shoulder belts. If the effectiveness of two-point belts is actually in the upper part of the range estimated by DOT, then the relative advantage of motorized shoulder belts would be even larger.

The next question is, how do the fatality reductions expected from the best automatic belt systems compare with those expected from air bags? Again, the answer depends on the levels of manual belt use achieved in cars with air bags. If 90 percent belt use could be achieved in air bag equipped cars, then about 48 percent of the fatalities could be prevented, according to DOT estimates. As

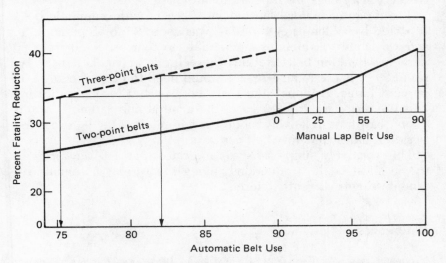

Figure 4-A-2   Comparative Reductions in Fatalities for Three-Point Automatic Belts and Two-Point Automatic Belts with Manual
Lap Belt Use of 25 and 55 percent. Based on midpoint of
effectiveness range (40-50 percent) estimated for three-
point belts and lowest effectiveness (35 percent) estimated
for two-point belts.

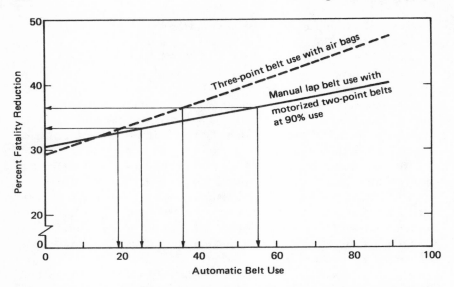

Figure 4-A-3   Comparative Reductions in Fatalities from Air Bags and
                Motorized Two-Point Belts for Different Levels of Manual
                Belt Use.

Figure 4–A–3 shows, at this high belt use level, the lifesaving benefits of air bags are superior to automatic belts.

The range of manual lap belt use in cars with automatic belts reported by Williams et al. (1987) was about 25 to 55 percent. To achieve fatality reductions comparable to that expected from 90 percent shoulder belt use and these levels of lap belt use, lap shoulder belt use in air bag cars would need to be in the 20 to 35 percent range. Although there are no reported results indicating belt use levels in air bag cars in the general population, it seems likely that these relatively modest levels could easily be exceeded in states with mandatory belt use laws.

This relatively simple analysis indicates that air bags promise the greatest fatality reductions among the various automatic restraint designs currently offered.

References

National Highway Traffic Safety Administration. 1984. *Final Regulatory Impact Analysis: Amendment to Federal Motor Vehicle Safety Standard 208*. Washington, D.C.: U.S. Dept. of Transportation.

WILLIAMS, A. F., WELLS, J. K., LUND, A. K., and TEED, N. 1987. "Observed Use of Automatic Seat Belts in 1987 Cars." Washington, D.C.: Insurance Institute for Highway Safety.

p 90'

111 - 15

9213

U.S.

~~951~~

6314

COMMENTS BY JOHN VERSACE

John Graham and Max Henrion's work is in the tradition of a number of restraint benefit estimations. The basic effectiveness figures used as inputs by Graham and Henrion were drawn from NHTSA's 1984 "Regulatory Impact Analysis" (Docket 74–14; N36), which was in turn a more or less consensual synthesis of the estimates various parties, including we, had developed over the years. All these efforts are aimed at estimating the future effect of things that have not much been done before and are therefore subject to considerable uncertainty.

The current effort differs from previous ones in at least two ways. First, this study uses credibility distributions for each of the factors making up the model, with Monte Carlo selection of values from those distributions to arrive at Bayesian credibility estimates for the solution. Second, it starts with a more general, aggregative perspective rather than a piecewise build-up from individual accident types. Some of the earlier efforts started with much more highly segmented partitions of the exposure universe: direction of force (crash type) by intensity of force by seated position, etc. For each of several assumptions about alternative restraints, the cells of such tables were filled with point estimates of effectiveness— some purely subjective, some based on biomechanical modeling, some based on laboratory or accident data. These piecewise effectiveness estimates were aggregated using relative frequency weightings taken from the accident data to yield the overall estimates, which in turn were multiplied by the point estimates of usage. The value in such segmentation is that the cause-effect nature of the crash event is easier to conceptualize when the circumstances are severely delimited; hence, there is more confidence the estimates are accurate.

The model did not take into account all the ways discretionary belt use figures into the various restraint configurations. All air bag systems today, and into the foreseeable future, are supplemental systems: they accompany a voluntary three-point belt. And most two-point passive belt systems also provide a voluntary lap belt. Nevertheless, the main value of this study is in what it will stimulate rather than in its findings. It sets forth an appealing approach that is unfamiliar to many in the traffic safety analysis field, and particularly to those who have made estimates of risk/benefit for restraints.

Input Variables

There are probably some better estimates for the input variables in Table 4–1. For example, the 50 percent fatality reduction effectiveness input (at the upper end) for the two-point "shoulder belt/knee pads" without lap belt is the same as for the three-point "lap/shoulder belt," an equivalence we would expect if lap belts were used. Performance of the two-point shoulder belt/knee pads arrangement without the lap belt may be equal or even superior to the three-point in *frontal* collisions. These cars pass the government's required crash tests without the lap belt. But effectiveness without the lap belt is not as well known for real-world *nonfrontal* collisions. NHTSA's study of VW undifferentiated field experience showed a considerable net advantage of the two-point arrangement (lap belts were not provided) but largely because of the very high usage. In actual practice the effectiveness may not be very different because where the lap belt is provided, as in the Ford Escort, its usage already has been observed to be 30 to 40 percent or so. The same consideration applies to the air bag fatality effectiveness estimate, excepting that here it may be too low; belt use should be factored into this, too. Consider that in the Ford Tempo air bag fleet there was 87 percent use of the accompanying three-point belt in the 175 deployment crashes to date. While that may not be representative of the eventual public usage, it cannot be neglected. Whether the effectiveness estimates should be made a function of belt use or separate effectiveness estimates made for the use and nonuse cases and then summed, is a methodological choice.

The injury effectiveness figures in Table 4–1 are all larger than the corresponding fatality effectiveness figures. Despite whether that is so for other restraints, there are some unknowns about air bag injury performance without belts: We would expect there to be fewer of the more severe but much less frequent injuries, particularly injuries to the face and head—the kind that are hard to eliminate with belts alone in the very severe, frontal crashes. On the other hand, the air bag does not deploy for the very much greater number of collisions at fixed barrier speeds of about 12 mph or less—about like striking a parked car at 25 mph. So there may be more of the less severe injuries rather than fewer, as compared to belt wearing. Furthermore, there is a not well understood potential risk due to the air bag itself striking out-of-position occupants (the unrestrained child or adult pitching forth under severe braking, or those with the seat up close). At this stage, the net effect of these three considerations is just not known.

The usage estimates in Table 4–1 might be raised. For the three-point "manual lap/shoulder belt," the three percentages for V may be more like 15, 25, and 35, or more. Strong laws can eventually lead to 90 percent or more use, like in the United Kingdom and West Germany. Although it is true that usage has been less in accident cases than in the public at large, those observations were made at a time when overall usage was very low. Use of the detachable, three-point automatic belt system has been observed to be rather greater than is shown in Table 4–1, perhaps by as much as 20 percentage points. For the two-point motorized passive belt restraints, the usage (and effectiveness) figures really need to be redone to take into account at least 30 to 40 percent on current lap belt use. The upper percentile for the fraction of cars in states allowing "voluntary" use is no longer as high as the 50 percent shown. After all, over 80 percent of the U.S. population now live in states with such laws. And that is likely to have some spillover effect in no-law states.

It may be surprising to some that equipment costs also tend to be uncertain, even for manufacturers. It is hard to know precisely how much things are going to cost in the future, especially if they are something with little if any history. Saying that, here are some opinions about the cost estimates in Table 4–1. "Manual" cost figures are probably about right. "Motorized" restraint figures are probably too low by $100. "Detachable" restraint estimates are probably more than $100 too low. "Twin air bags" figures are too low by perhaps as much as a couple hundred dollars at the low end and maybe $500 at the high end. What a supplier may report as the cost to provide parts it is not yet manufacturing (or has not even built the plants to do so) cannot be too reliable. Even if it were, it is not all the cost. System cost also includes the cost of knee bolsters and all the other vehicle modifications to accommodate the system plus extra test and engineering and assembly expenses. How much of this additional cost can be relieved in the long run is still open to debate.

Another thing to consider in Table 4–1 is the "base case death rate." Presumably, the rates are taken as 10-year rates, because the stated rate of 19.3 per 10,000 would otherwise be too large by a factor of 10. But that is not clear, as earlier in the paper it is stated that the base case fatalities and operating costs are distributed over a 15-year vehicle life using R. L. Polk survival data. (For simplicity of expression, we usually refer to these rates in per million form: e.g., 193 per million car-years.)

Results

The results of the analysis, presented in Tables 4–3 to 4–5, must reflect some of the considerations mentioned above. The lives-saved estimates for two-point "motorized" belts are probably high because the input effectiveness was too high. However, it might converge toward this if account were taken of the probable level of lap belt use. The three-point "detachable" result is probably underestimated, because of the overly small usage values postulated. To the extent that injuries are included in these figures, as "fractions" of fatalities, air bag injuries—because they are more or less unknown as per earlier comments—will likely make these results less reliable. The study also includes an interesting analysis of the relative contribution of input variables to final results, by means of rank correlations between them, although the exact methodology is not clear in the draft report. The findings that uncertainty about the input values for effectiveness and for the economic value of lifesaving are the major sources of output uncertainty might also change as some of the input estimates are changed.

There remains the fundamental conundrum about scaling the disutility of injury. Can any number of minor injuries equal a fatality? What is the proper measure of benefit—lives saved or travel achieved? Are lives saved a benefit or are they societal costs averted, or does that distinction matter? A former NHTSA counsel (Dyson, 1975) asked an interesting question: Why is loss of future earnings and other product a *societal* loss, since insurance replaces much of the loss and the unfortunate victim is replaced in the economy by someone else?

Graham and Henrion's conclusion that "Precise answers to these questions must await the large scale field test of air bags that is now being launched" is exactly the point. The fact is, we really don't know with any certainty what is going to happen when scores of millions are buckling up and there are millions of air bag cars out there. One of the problems in the eventual assessment of actual accident experience is in the development of a better methodology for scaling of injury, not to mention the accurate collecting of such data. Considering the similarity of the effectiveness estimates among the various restraint systems, it may be very difficult to show any differential effect on life saving in noisy, real-world data. The pattern of injury saving may be more discriminatory, providing that kind of data can be accurately obtained to begin with. This could be a challenge to those in the accident data field.

Whether cost-benefit studies like this are ultimately applicable to policies that involve death and injury—certainly they cannot be determinative—the application of the credibility of estimates methodology to the study of safety is to many of us an unfamiliar but very interesting approach that should be given serious consideration.

Reference

R. B. DYSON. 1975. "Safety versus Savings: An Essay on the Fallacy of Economic Costs of Accidents," May 15.

Chapter 5

MINIMUM LEGAL DRINKING AGES AND HIGHWAY SAFETY: A METHODOLOGICAL CRITIQUE

by Steven Garber

Introduction

During the early 1970s many states lowered their minimum legal drinking ages (MLDAs), but since the late 1970s the trend has been in the opposite direction. These policy changes provide unusual opportunities for policy analysis, and numerous empirical studies of the effects of both lowering and raising MLDAs have been conducted. In fact, it appears that studies of the effects of lowering MLDAs had considerable impact on the congressional debate that resulted in legislation aimed at a national, uniform MLDA of 21 years.

Empirical literature on the highway safety impacts of MLDA policies has been surveyed by Whitehead (1980); Wagenaar (1983, Ch. 3); GAO (1987); and Donelson, Beirness, and Mayhew (1987). Each is focused primarily on the question: Based on the available evidence, how effective are MLDAs in promoting highway safety? This emphasis reflects the important objective of informing today's policy decisions. In contrast, the present review is aimed at improving the scientific quality of the research that will inform

I thank Heather Campbell, John D. Graham, and Kathryn Shaw for helpful comments on a previous draft.

116

policy decisions years in the future—another important objective. Accordingly, the focus here is methodological. Moreover, since the methods critiqued here in the context of the MLDA literature are also widely employed in the highway safety literature at large, various criticisms and recommendations pertain more broadly than the title of this chapter might suggest.

Empirical studies have been conducted by individuals trained in various research traditions, including economics, engineering, psychology, and statistics. Apparently as a result, the empirical literature contains studies based on very different methods, thus providing substantial grist for a methodological review. Four general approaches are prominent: two that attempt "statistical control" and two that attempt control by "quasi-experimental design." Each is described and evaluated.

Despite the fact that some approaches seem far more promising than others, constructive suggestions are offered for improving the implementation of each. There are at least three reasons for doing so. First, even the methods that seem generally less promising may be appropriate in some instances (due to factors such as data availability, time constraints on the analyst, and the sophistication of the client or intended audience). Second, as emphasized below, the promise of a particular approach in a particular context depends on subtle issues that can be resolved only with expertise not possessed by the author. Finally, it is expected that each of the approaches will continue to be used, appropriate or not!

Two caveats seem appropriate. First, the author has been trained primarily as an economist and econometrician. As a result, he is more familiar with (1) economic than with competing perspectives on human behavior; and (2) methods of statistical control than with control by quasi-experimental design. Because this survey is intended to be useful to researchers from all of the traditions represented in the literature, an attempt is made to convey the perspective and to provide and explain the essential jargon from each field. It is likely, however, that this effort is more successful for economists, with whom the author is more experienced in communicating. Second, while much literature has been reviewed, some empirical studies of the highway safety impacts of MLDA have not. Most obviously underrepresented are unpublished studies and early studies of the effects of decreasing MLDAs. All indications from the literature reviewed, especially the recent surveys cited above, are, however, that the studies not reviewed involve no methods fundamentally different from those reviewed.

In the next section, the decision problem of an idealized policymaker is briefly considered. This facilitates the exposition of various general issues relevant to enhancing the usefulness of future studies and provides a foundation for the analyses that follow. One issue raised in the next section—controlling for other factors—is fundamental and merits extensive consideration. The remainder of the chapter emphasizes this issue.

The chapter next describes the four general approaches to control. Motivations offered in the literature for choices of general method and means of implementation are also reviewed. The next section is the heart of the chapter; it critiques each approach and selected studies applying them. In particular, the focus is on the development of the conditions under which each method would succeed in isolating the policy-relevant component of an observed highway safety outcome. The overriding objective is to raise and clarify important methodological issues. Resolution of many of these requires attention by highway safety specialists. The chapter concludes with some general comments concerning promising and less promising research strategies.

Implications of Decision Analysis for Empirical Analysis

Empirical studies of the effects of MLDAs are generally under-taken to inform policy, but the links between the empirical analysis and the decision problem of the policymaker are generally not made explicit. While this may reflect a desire not to restrict the potential audience (e.g., among policymakers or interest groups facing diverse decision problems), failure to make the decision context explicit also has disadvantages. These include the failure to address the types of policy decisions for which the reported estimates are relevant and failure to appreciate methodological prescriptions suggested by a general decision-theoretic perspective. In this section aspects of an idealized decision problem are considered in order to raise various concerns relevant to enhancing the usefulness of future empirical studies. Many of these issues are illustrated in subsequent discussions of selected empirical studies of MLDA and highway safety.

Consider a specific policy proposal aimed at improved highway safety. Let the elements of the vector z contain variables that would be directly manipulated in the event that the policy is adopted. The proposed policy would involve changing (one or more of the elements of) z from some *status quo* level, z^0 say, to z^1. The major benefits would include reductions in fatalities, injuries, property damage, and medical care costs. Collect meas-ures of such outcomes in the $S \times 1$ vector y. The extent of the benefits attributable to the policy depends on the quantitative impacts of changes in the elements of z on the elements of y. These impacts are assumed to depend on the functions:

$$y_s = f_s(z; x) \quad s = 1,2,...S, \qquad (5.1)$$

where: y_s = the level of the sth highway safety outcome, and x is a $K \times 1$ vector containing the variables that affect highway safety outcomes but are not under the control of the policymaker.

The elements of x might include measures of climate, terrain, driving activity (perhaps disaggregated by times of the day and ages and driving experience of drivers), "sociocultural setting" (see, Wagenaar, 1983, p. 122), and drinking "sentiment" (Saffer and Grossman, 1987a,b). This vector would also include variables representing highway safety policies other than those directly manipulated by the proposed policy. In the case of an evaluation of a proposal to change MLDA policy, the vector x might include measures of laws and enforcement efforts in areas such as speed limits, drunken driving, seat belt usage, and alcohol taxes.

The S functions in (5.1) represent abstractly the opportunities of the policymaker to affect the highway safety outcomes by changing policies. Explicit attention to the variables x reflects the fact that observed changes in highway safety outcomes after changes in z will, in general, be attributable in part to factors not under the control of the policymaker. The challenge in empirical policy evaluation is to isolate the components of the changes in y that are relevant for policy—those components which are meaningfully viewed as being caused by the policy changes. From a statistical point of view, interest would focus on the joint distribution of (or empirical associations between) z and y conditional on (or holding constant) the variables in x. The various means by which researchers have attempted to hold such factors constant are the focus of the following two sections.

In evaluating a policy proposal, ideally one would compare its benefits and costs in comparable units of measurement. Generally, quantification in terms of dollars is convenient. Value judgments vary widely concerning the social (dollar) value of averting highway fatalities or injuries, however. Thus quantification of benefits in terms of fatalities and injuries avoided (rather than dollars) seems appropriate. The role for policy analysis on the cost side seems even more limited. These costs (such as limitation of individual freedom—see Wagenaar, 1983, Ch. 6, and Donelson, Beirness, and Mayhew, 1987, pp. 117–22, for other examples) defy useful quantification in any units of measurement. Therefore, in the case of a proposal to change MLDA policy, policy analysis seems best focused on providing information about the functions in (5.1). Ideally, policymakers would use this information about public health benefits, in combination with their value judgments about the social value of lifesaving, individual freedom, etc., to make a decision.

The functions in (5.1) highlight a number of issues bearing on the information that an idealized decisionmaker would desire from a policy analyst. First, various highway safety outcomes are of concern. In principle, the decisionmaker would want, for example, separate estimates of fatalities and injuries averted by the proposed policy (since these would be valued differently). Analysis of numbers of crashes (i.e., with fatal and nonfatal crashes simply aggregated, and thus treated as equivalent), which may make it easier to detect a public health benefit of MLDA policies (see Wagenaar, 1983, pp. 41, 102), is unattractive from this point of view. Demonstration of the *existence* of safety benefits, which preoccupies many of the researchers in this area, is a very modest objective. Estimates of the *extent* of benefits in policy-relevant units of measurement would generally be desired for decisionmaking, at least by our idealized policymaker.

Second, MLDA policies have various dimensions, and failure to consider this can contribute to inappropriate interpretation of results. For example, the results of Naor and Nashold (1975), it seems, have been interpreted by some as indicating that "lowering MLDAs" would have no public health costs. But they studied a rather special "lowering of MLDA": beer had been legally available to 18-year-olds *before* the policy change affecting their data, which merely lowered the MLDA for other beverages to 18 (see Wagenaar, 1983, p. 19). While often it is impractical to distinguish dimensions of MLDA policy empirically because of lack of data or lack of independent variation in various elements of z, the results must then be interpreted accordingly. Cook and Tauchen (1984, p. 179) provide a nice example of appropriate interpretation of the coefficient of a variable that is implicitly measuring (because of colinearity) various dimensions of MLDA policy.

Third, the effects of changes in the elements of z on the elements of y depend in principle on the levels of the variables in x. Such "interactions" may be central to useful interpretation of results for policy purposes. For example, the effectiveness of a particular change in MLDA policy is likely to depend substantially on the price of alcohol, the purchasing power of youths, drunken driving laws and their enforcement, and seat belt usage rates. Such considerations may be critical in understanding differences in estimated effectiveness levels of specific MLDA policies implemented at distinct times or in distinct locales. Moreover, looking beyond the narrow question of MLDA policy, such interactions may be essential to any reliable characterization of the optimal mix of highway safety policies.

A final issue pertains to the nature of the statistical information generated by empirical studies of MLDA. All of these studies are conducted within the classical (frequentist, sampling theory) framework. But, the results of classical statistical analysis are not well connected to the needs of a decisionmaker. It would be very helpful if empirical results could be used to address questions such as, what is the probability that the proposed policy will avert more than 1,000 deaths? But such questions are not meaningful within the classical framework, in which probability cannot be interpreted subjectively (as in the question) as a degree of belief. Bayesian statistical analysis is ideally suited for decisionmaking, but it seems very likely that classical analyses will remain predominant.

This being the case, it is especially important to avoid some very common misunderstandings in the interpretation of classical hypothesis tests. First, failure to reject the hypothesis of no highway safety impacts does not imply that the best estimate of the effect is zero. This very common, but inappropriate, "inference" is implicit in various of the studies reviewed here.

Second, and more subtle, is the related fact that classical significance levels (p-values) generally cannot be sensibly interpreted as probabilities that the null hypothesis is correct. Casella and Berger (1987) and Berger and Selke (1987) are recent analyses of the conditions under which p-values can be interpreted as Bayesian posterior probabilities of the null hypothesis. These conditions are very restrictive, and p-values can differ dramatically from Bayesian posterior probabilities. (A very useful discussion of this issue, aimed primarily at psychologists, is contained in Oakes, 1986.)

For example, suppose a researcher rejects the null hypothesis that the effect of a policy is 1,000 lives saved in favor of the hypothesis that the effect is greater than 1,000, with a p-value of .03. This does not allow one to conclude that the probability that the effect is no greater than 1,000 is .03 or any other particular number. Classical p-values reflect not only the closeness of the true parameter value to some hypothesized value, but also the amount of information contained in the data. Hypotheses that are for all practical purposes correct (e.g., true effect is 1,001 lives saved and the null hypothesis is 1,000 lives saved) may be rejected confidently if sufficient data are available. Conversely, hypotheses that are dramatically incorrect will not be rejected if sufficiently little data are available.

In the next section, four general approaches to holding other relevant factors constant are described. These approaches and selected studies employing them are then critiqued. Other points raised above are illustrated in the course of critiquing various studies.

Four General Approaches to Holding Other Factors Constant: Description

The parameters of interest to the policymaker are taken to be the (partial) derivatives of the expected values of the safety outcomes (y_s) with respect to changes in MLDAs (z) holding constant the other determinants of y_s (x). Various means of attempting to "hold x constant" have been used in the empirical literature on the highway safety impacts of MLDA policies. Each involves one of four conceptually distinct general approaches. The first two are attempts to hold other factors constant *statistically* and the last two by *quasi-experimental design*. Primary objectives here are to clarify the conditions under which each of these approaches will succeed in isolating the effects of changes in MLDA policies and thereby to facilitate exploration of the implications of these conditions.

In the remainder of this section each approach is described, and rationales offered by their adherents are reported. Analyses and critiques are reserved for the following section, where each approach is interpreted formally in order to clarify the conditions under which it would allow isolation of the policy-relevant components of observed changes in highway safety outcomes. Judgments concerning the degree to which these conditions are approximated in various instances require highway safety expertise exceeding that possessed by the author. Thus in many instances the analysis goes only as far as posing questions that seem worthy of attention by specialists in the area. Answers to these questions, combined with the analyses offered below, are expected to provide a foundation for evaluation of the received empirical literature and design of future studies.

Method 1: Statistical Analysis Explicitly Controlling for Other Theoretical Causes *(Colon, 1984; Hoxie and Skinner, 1985, Model I; Asch and Levy, 1987a; Saffer and Grossman, 1987a, 1987b; Wilkinson, 1987)*

To many, a natural approach to controlling for other factors would be to (1) specify (by appeal to theory, previous empirical findings, or both) the appropriate elements of the vector **x**; (2) measure these factors; and (3) use these data in a (multivariate) statistical analysis designed to "hold constant" their influences. Multiple regression analysis is well suited to such an endeavor, and a number of researchers have used multiple regression to study the effects of MLDA policies. In principle, it can be applied to cross-sectional data, time series data, or ("panel" or "pooled") data combining cross-sections and time series.

In most instances, highway safety outcomes—for example, fatality rates for particular age groups—are used as dependent variables. The independent variables are measures of MLDA policies and variables representing other theoretically relevant determinants of such outcomes. Interest centers on the estimated coefficient of the MLDA variable. Assuming that the other independent variables adequately capture—that is, hold constant statistically—the influences of all other relevant determinants of the highway safety outcome, the estimated coefficient of an MLDA variable can be interpreted as an estimate of the partial effect of a unit change in that variable on the expected value of the highway safety outcome.

For example, Hoxie and Skinner (1985, p. 11) write: "The problem is to isolate the effect of changes in MDA from all other influences on highway fatalities." They pool annual observations for the 50 states and the District of Columbia for each of the years 1975 to 1984. The dependent variable is fatalities involving 18- to 20-year-old drivers per population aged 18 to 20. The MLDA variable reflects *changes* from the previous year in policy with regard to purchase of beer of any alcoholic content, and is carefully constructed to reflect the age groups affected, the fraction of the year for which the new policy was in force, and grandfathering. They considered various regression specifications, employing as control variables proxies representing various conceptual determinants of the fatality outcome (see their Table 8). They present both ordinary and weighted least-squares estimates for their "Model I," which "is felt to be the best model that can be constructed . . . using only available socio-economic and activity driving [sic] data . . . in the sense of having theoretically important variables which are statistically significant and which explain more of the variation than other models" (p. 24). This specification includes as control variables (see p. 27) per capita consumption of malt beverages, fraction of vehicle miles traveled that are in rural areas, and the unemployment rate for all workers.

Asch and Levy (1987a) examine a cross-section of the 50 states observed in 1978. They describe their general strategy: "In effect, we introduce drinking age measures into conventional regression equations explaining traffic fatality rates . . ." (p. 182). They consider various fatality rates as dependent variables and various MLDA variables. Used as controls are variables "suggested by the existing traffic safety literature" (p. 182). In addition to being a relatively ambitious attempt to control explicitly for other causal factors, this study emphasizes the distinction between the effect of *youthful* use of alcohol (the target of MLDAs) and *inexperience* in drinking, which may be merely delayed by increasing MLDAs. They also consider empirically whether their results might be due to joint determination of fatalities and MLDA policy—that is, potential endogeneity of MLDA—and "border crossing" effects. With regard to the former issue, if MLDA policies are in part reactions to fatality rates, then this implies a causal link *from* fatalities *to* MLDA, and "simultaneous-equations bias" is thus of concern. (This statistical pitfall is sometimes characterized in terms of "feedback" from the dependent variable to an independent variable or in terms of "reverse causality.")

Saffer and Grossman (1987a) study motor vehicle death rates for ages 15 to 17, 18 to 20, and 21 to 24, pooling annual observations from 1975 to 1981 for each of the contiguous 48 states. At least three general features of this study deserve emphasis. The first is the evaluation of MLDA in conjunction with another policy that may be even more promising, in the cost-benefit sense, in reducing alcohol-related highway fatalities: increasing taxes on beer. Second, they are more explicit with regard to the theoretical underpinnings of their empirical specification than is typical of the MLDA literature, most notably in emphasizing determinants of alcohol consumption and in the use of the concept of "drinking sentiment." In addition, in the absence of a strong basis for preferring a single method, they implement (and report results for) alternative methods of controlling for some theoretical determinants.

Saffer and Grossman (1987b) analyze largely the same data, specifying and estimating a two-equation model in which mortality rates are jointly determined with MLDA. (Endogeneity of the legal drinking age is especially plausible during their sample period— 1975 to 1981—a period characterized by increases in MLDA that are believed to be largely a reaction to highway deaths.) This study employs the drinking sentiment construct in conjunction with another unobservable: pressure to pass a drinking age of 21, which is viewed as a function of drinking sentiment and, if the drinking age is not 21, the youth mortality rate.

Wilkinson (1987) also considers MLDA in conjunction with other policies, such as drunken driving enforcement levels, enforcement of speed limits, and closing times for drinking establishments, in a model in which MLDA is assumed to affect fatality rates indirectly through its effects on alcohol consumption levels. Like Saffer and Grossman (1987a,b), Wilkinson (1987) is unusually explicit concerning theoretical underpinnings of his empirical specification.

Method 2: Statistical Analysis with "Dummy-Variable Controls" (*Cook and Tauchen, 1984; Hoxie and Skinner, 1985, Model II; DuMouchel, Williams, and Zador, 1987; Asch and Levy, 1987b*)

Various studies attempt to hold constant statistically other relevant determinants of the highway safety outcome by using variables that do *not* explicitly represent theoretical causes of that outcome. Typically, these variables are dichotomous indicators distinguishing observations according to various dimensions. Hence the terminology—"dummy-variable controls." This method is generally applied to "pooled" or "panel" data—typically, a cross-section of times series. The specification widely used in the MLDA literature is often referred to as a "fixed effects" model and the estimation procedure as an "analysis of covariance" (see Judge et al., 1985, Ch. 13; or Maddala, 1977, Ch. 14).

For example, Cook and Tauchen (1984) used data for the 48 contiguous states for each of the years from 1970 to 1977. Highway safety outcomes are used as the dependent variable. The independent variables are measures of MLDA policy and dummy variables allowing for a different regression intercept for each state and year. Hoxie and Skinner's approach (1985, Model II) is quite similar. Asch and Levy's (1987b) is also similar, but they incorporate variables representing experience in (legal) drinking as well.

DuMouchel, Williams and Zador (1987) jointly analyzed data with three observational dimensions: each observation pertained to drivers of one of nine particular ages (16 to 24) in one of the 48 contiguous states in one of the years 1975 to 1984. They regressed the logarithm of the number of "driver fatal involvements" for a particular driver age in a particular state in a particular year on (1) an MLDA variable (the proportion of this year for which individuals of this age were allowed to purchase alcohol in this state); (2) a variable reflecting the state population of individuals of this age in this year; (3) many dummy variables distinguishing state-age pairs and state-year pairs; (4) a single variable allowing for a particular form of age-year interactions; and (5) (in some of their analyses) variables constructed to examine "whether the first year of being legally allowed to purchase alcohol is especially hazardous" (pp. 262–63).

Cook and Tauchen (1984) decline to employ control variables explicitly linked to theory, explaining (p. 177) that:

> *A multivariate analysis of the determinants of state auto fatality rates, with MLDA and all other important determinants as independent variables, could conceivably . . . generate a reliable estimate of the MLDA effect from cross-section data. Results of this type of analysis tend to be sensitive to specification errors, however.*

They address another method popular in the MLDA literature when they write (p. 177): "The interrupted time-series technique can be used to assess the impact of MLDA change in each jurisdiction separately, but it is a cumbersome tool for analyzing the impact of MLDAs from a national perspective." Their use of state dummies is addressed on page 176: ". . . state fatality rates differ widely for reasons that tend to persist over time—road conditions, average distance traveled by residents each year, traffic law enforcement efforts, drinking practices, and so forth." With regard to the time dummies, they refer (p. 178) to "the 'year' effect, which captures movements in national variables such as business conditions and the price of fuel."

Hoxie and Skinner (1985) motivate their Model II by concern about omitted-variable bias in Model I. They write: "To protect against the effects of an omitted variable, dummy variables are used to test and account for unexplained variation associated with either state or year." Asch and Levy (1987b, pp. 6–7) explain their use of state and year dummy variables this way: "*State-specific effects* control for variation in population characteristics, traffic safety enforcement efforts, and other intrinsic distinctions. *Calendar-time* effects control for factors such as nationwide trends in traffic fatality experience."

DuMouchel, Williams, and Zador (1987) adopt an even more elaborate means of attempting to hold other factors constant, which is made feasible by their pooling across age groups as well as states and years. In their words (p. 259): "This model is similar in spirit to that of Cook and Tauchen. . . . The more complex model used here is intended to protect against several sources of bias. . . . This model . . . allows the state effects to vary by age, allows the year effects to vary by state. . . ." Thus, they choose to use dummy variables to control for other factors, but they seem doubtful that state and year dummies alone provide adequate controls.

Method 3: Simple Paired Comparisons (Naor and Nashold, 1975; Ferreira and Sicherman, 1976; Hingson et al., 1983; Williams et al., 1983; Males, 1986; Hoskin, Yalung-Mathews, and Carraro, 1986)

Another method of attempting to hold other factors constant is well known in the "quasi-experimental design" literature: comparing changes in highway safety outcomes, before and after a change in MLDA policy, between two situations, one believed sensitive and the other insensitive to a change in MLDA policy. The latter is viewed as a "control" or "comparison" group. Comparison groups that have been used include (1) states that didn't change their MLDA policy; (2) age groups not directly affected by the change in MLDA policy; and (3) types of accidents that are believed to be relatively insensitive to the change in MLDA policy.

Cook and Campbell (1979) distinguish between two basic reasons that an outcome may be insensitive to a "treatment" (in our context, a change in MLDA policy): (1) there was no treatment ("nonequivalent no-treatment control group"); and (2) the treatment is believed to be irrelevant to a particular outcome ("nonequivalent dependent variables"). Comparison states provide an example of the former, and comparison age groups or types of crashes within the state that changed its MLDA policy exemplify the latter.

For example, consider a state that changes the legal status of 18- to 20-year-olds with regard to the purchase of alcohol. In order to evaluate the effect of this change in MLDA policy, one might compare differences in fatality rates of 18- to 20-year-olds in a particular state before and after that state changed its MLDA to the corresponding change in fatality rates for a (comparison) state that did not change its MLDA. Alternatively, one might compare within the state that changed its MLDA differences in fatality rates of 18- to 20-year-olds (before and after the policy change) to the corresponding differences in fatality rates for an age group whose legal status with regard to alcohol purchase was unaffected by the change in MLDA, often chosen as 21- to 24-year-olds. Finally, since daytime crash fatalities are less likely to involve alcohol than nighttime crash fatalities—and, thus, daytime fatal crashes may be substantially less sensitive to MLDA policies than are nighttime fatal crashes—the relative levels of daytime and nighttime fatalities might be compared before and after a state changes its MLDA. Combinations of these ideas have also been employed (e.g., see the discussion below of Males, 1986). In principle, the effect of other factors on these fatality rates may be effectively controlled because these factors might "net out" in making the comparison.

A particularly prominent example of this approach is Williams et al. (1983). They studied nine states that increased their MLDAs between September 1, 1976 and January 1, 1980. Each of these states was paired with a "comparison state." The choice of comparison states is explained this way: "Comparison states were chosen on the basis of geographic proximity to the law-change states and comparability of law-change states with respect to numbers of crash fatalities" (p. 170). Williams (1986, p. 213) explains that comparison states were used (in Williams et al., 1983) to "rule out the possibility that changes observed in youthful crash involvement were merely part of a regional trend." Williams et al. (1983) also made comparisons across age groups, and in this regard Williams (1986, p. 213) writes that these comparisons were used to "rule out the possibility that changes observed in age groups covered by the laws were part of a trend occurring at other ages as well."

Males (1986, p. 193) considers 14 pairs of states, writing: "The matches, where possible, have similar numbers of fatal crashes." He compares across paired states the ratios within states of fatal crashes involving a driver from an age group directly affected by the change in MLDA policy to fatal crashes involving drivers aged 21 to 24. Males (1986, p. 194) explains his use of these "fatal crash ratios" (FCRs) in a way that directly addresses causal factors that he is attempting thereby to hold constant:

> The FCR, as opposed to raw numbers of fatalities or fatality rate, is chosen to eliminate state-specific factors other than MLPA increases. Factors such as the state's economy, weather, highway conditions, average driver speeds, miles driven per driver, law enforcement, tougher drunk driving laws, and so on would presumably affect drivers ages twenty-one to twenty-four in a manner roughly equivalent to under-twenty-one drivers.

Hingson et al. (1983, p. 164), in which New York is used as a comparison state for Massachusetts, explains the choice this way: "At the time that Massachusetts raised its legal drinking age from 18 to 20, the two states had similar laws regarding age of driving licensure and penalties for driving while intoxicated. . . . Being contiguous, the two states also have roughly similar weather patterns." Finally, Donelson, Beirness, and Mayhew (1987, p. 56), in a comprehensive, critical review of the empirical literature, write: "The selection of a same age-control group from another jurisdiction . . . should be done based on the initial comparability of drinking practices, driving patterns, accident rates, enforcement practices, traffic laws, and regulations pertaining to young drivers, etc."

Method 4: Paired Comparisons Employing Statistical Projection *(Ferreira and Sicherman, 1976; various studies by Douglass and others described in Douglass, 1980; Wagenaar, 1982, 1983, 1986; and Wagenaar and Maybee, 1986)*

In this second approach to control by quasi-experimental design, the paired comparisons are based on discrepancies between observed outcomes and their *projected* levels in the absence of a policy intervention (such as a change in MLDA policy), rather than their *observed* levels *before* the intervention (as in the case of "simple paired comparisons"). Wagenaar (1983, pp. 115–16) indicates that the purpose of projecting is to guard against the possibility that the "postintervention observations were simply the continuation of a preintervention maturational trend" and the use of comparison groups is to guard against "history, a contemporaneous event that may have caused the observed effects." ("History" and "maturation" are jargon from the quasi-experimental design literature.) With regard to the use of other age and other state comparison groups, Wagenaar (1983, p. 116) writes : "Contemporaneous historical events would most likely affect all age groups in all four states." The projections employ more or less detailed time series data on highway safety outcomes prior to the change in MLDA policy, which enables the use of statistical extrapolation methods.

The basic idea is that an "intervention," such as a change in MLDA policy, that has a substantial impact on a highway safety outcome, y, should alter noticeably the time path of y at the time that the policy intervention is implemented. (Hence, the terminology "interrupted time series," which is common in the quasi-experimental design literature.) Often, methods are applied using data only for y, coupled with knowledge about the timing of the intervention(s) and assumptions about the form (but not magnitude) of the effect of the intervention(s). The objective is to characterize usefully the time series behavior of y from before the intervention and thereby enable decomposition of the postintervention levels of y into those parts reflecting the continuation or extrapolation of the preintervention time series process and those parts that are to be attributed to the intervention, if the comparisons suggest that such an interpretation is warranted.

Technical difficulties involve the specification and estimation of times series processes allowing for fairly elaborate patterns reflecting (most often) "trend" and "seasonality." The nature of these patterns is also viewed by Wagenaar (1983, p. 39) as relevant to the choice of comparison jurisdictions: "New York and Pennsylvania were chosen for comparison purposes because the climate and cyclical (seasonal) patterns in crash involvement were similar to those of Maine and Michigan."

In many univariate time series analyses, attention is restricted to the class of stochastic processes known as ARIMA processes, and Wagenaar works within that class as well. In particular, Wagenaar employs techniques recommended by Box and Tiao (1975) and Box and Jenkins (1976), which he contends (Wagenaar, 1983, p. 125) are "the best currently available for the analysis of time-series quasi-experiments." Cook and Campbell (1979, p. 213) and Donelson, Beirness, and Mayhew (1987, p. 58) also enthusiastically endorse this approach.

Wagenaar (1983, Appendix B) explains his application of these methods and provides some hints concerning why he chose to use them. First, he argues (p. 125) that "ordinary least-squares regression and other commonly used statistical procedures could not be used for this study because they assume independent observations." This argument, which echoes that of McCain and McCleary (1979, pp. 234–35), is unpersuasive. For example, regression analysis allowing for dependence (e.g., generalized least-squares or maximum-likelihood estimation assuming serially correlated disturbances) is hardly esoteric and might well be recommended if one's only concern is the inappropriateness of ordinary least-squares with dependent observations.

More interesting, and more difficult to dismiss, is the motivation implicit in Wagenaar (1983, p. 126): "It is important to realize that the ARIMA model is not based on a theory of the causes of the dependent series. It is a model to describe the nature of the ongoing regularities in the series caused by any number of (most likely unidentified) causes." The implication seems to be that theoretical determination of the elements of the vector x is infeasible; thus measurement and explicit control of them is out of the question.

Four General Approaches to Holding Other Factors Constant: Analysis and Critique

Four approaches have been described, and each may be useful. Interest thus centers on the advantages and disadvantages of a particular approach in a particular setting, and how application of each approach may be improved. However, the literature provides sparse guidance in these regards: generally, little explanation is offered for a choice of methods. Moreover, methods are more often rationalized on the basis of claimed weaknesses of the alternatives than on the strengths of method adopted, and readers are almost never helped to appreciate potential pitfalls of the method used. Explicit attention to such issues seems necessary, however, to judge the reliability of received estimates and to aid researchers in designing future studies.

In this section the four approaches are examined critically. The primary objective is clarification of the conditions under which each approach would succeed in "holding other relevant factors constant," thus allowing isolation of policy-relevant empirical associations between MLDA policies and traffic safety outcomes. Appreciation of these conditions is prerequisite to judging the extent to which alternative research strategies are likely to be appropriate, and how best to implement them in a particular context. In various instances, the extent to which these conditions are approximated is a difficult question that can be satisfactorily addressed only with considerable infusions of detailed knowledge of highway safety phenomena. Thus, in many instances the contribution here is restricted to the framing of issues and posing of questions that merit careful consideration by highway safety experts.

Major themes of this section are: (1) *any* statistical method can be misapplied and contribute to ill-advised policies; (2) appreciation of the strengths and weaknesses of alternative methods is required for satisfactory evaluation or application; and (3) explicit consideration of the *theoretical* determinants of the outcomes of interest is required to develop appreciation for these strengths and weaknesses.

The word "theory" means various things to various people. To clarify, the following *(Webster's Seventh New Collegiate Dictionary)* definitions are enumerated: "a plausible or scientifically acceptable general principle or body of principles offered to explain phenomena," "a hypothesis assumed for the sake of argument or investigation," and "abstract thought." When the words "theory," "theoretical," etc., are used below, all three of these connotations are implied.

Rigorous analysis of the strengths and weaknesses of the various approaches require an explicit characterization of the process that generated the data on a highway safety outcome, y. *For purposes of analysis*, assume that the data-generating process (DGP) is:

$$y_i = z_i'\gamma + x_i'\beta + \epsilon_i \qquad (5.2)$$

where i indexes observations; y_i is a particular highway safety outcome for observational-unit i; z_i is a vector of variables characterizing the MLDA policy in i; x_i is a vector of other variables assumed to affect y_i; ϵ_i represents the determinants of y that are usefully viewed as "random" or unsystematic (in particular, ϵ is assumed mean-independent of $[z, x]$); and β and γ are vectors of parameters. The elements of γ are the parameters of policy interest and are interpreted as the partial derivatives of the expected value of y_i with respect to the elements of z_i (i.e., the dimensions of MLDA policy) holding constant other determinants of y_i. The variables in x_i are viewed (for purposes of policy evaluation) as "control" or "confounding" variables, and their coefficients, β, are not of direct policy interest.

Note, in particular, that the *general* DGP (5.2) is not viewed as the "true" process. Various *specific* DGPs result from (5.2) and distinct specifications of the elements of z and x. For such a specific DGP to be interesting, it need "merely" be an abstract, but to some people plausible, representation that some would be willing to entertain for purposes of investigation. Different researchers will disagree about the relative usefulness of various specific DGPs. In the present context, disagreement is assumed to be restricted to specification of the elements of the vectors z and x, and the discussion and analysis are structured to accommodate disagreements about this issue. Such disagreements are the fundamental reason that much of the analysis stops short of an overall judgment: different plausible DGPs might lead to different judgments, and resolution thus requires explicit consideration of issues that engender controversy among highway safety experts.

Theoretical specification of the elements of the vectors z_i and x_i is difficult and controversial. Even if the elements of these vectors can be satisfactorily specified, measurement of these variables is likely to be very difficult. Thus (5.2) is not viewed as providing a direct prescription concerning how to estimate γ, which appears to be very challenging. Rather, (5.2) is used to interpret the various approaches found in the literature in order to clarify the settings in which each is likely to be more or less useful.

Method 1: Statistical Analysis Explicitly Controlling for Other Theoretical Causes

These studies are viewed as attempts to implement specific versions of (5.2) directly. Any such attempt, however, is likely to be controversial. Controversy would reflect differences in theoretical perspectives (i.e., the appropriate *conceptualizations* of the vectors z and, especially, x) and measurement difficulties (i.e., the empirical implementation of these concepts). Regression is the predom-

inant statistical tool used by economists, and econometrics textbooks contain extensive discussions of pitfalls. These include
statistical consequences of various forms of "misspecification," any
one of which implies that standard regression estimators of the
elements of γ have no desirable sampling properties (and, thus,
have nothing to recommend them from the point of view of
classical statistics). Studies of MLDA involving explicit statistical
control of other relevant determinants are a relatively recent
addition to the literature, and there is room for improvement. The
discussion that follows focuses on general issues that warrant
attention.

The Hoxie and Skinner (1985) analysis raises two issues of
general concern. The first is a specification issue about which there
seems to be considerable confusion in the MLDA literature. In
particular, in their specifications the MLDA variable refers to
changes in policy, and the dependent variable refers to *levels* of
fatality rates. Such specifications seem to be of quite limited
interest. Some speculation, based in part on Donelson, Beirness,
and Mayhew (1987, p. 57), is useful here for expository purposes.
It seems that the MLDA variable is specified in terms of changes
because the policy question is generally framed in terms of the
effects of a proposed change. More tentatively, the dependent
variable is expressed in terms of fatality rates, rather than the
change in fatality rate, because fatalities are the major policy
concern. This type of approach to specification, however, ignores
what many would view as an overriding specification principle: the
regression equation is to express most sensibly one's theoretical
view of the causal process determining the dependent variable.

Bluntly, it seems to make much more sense to posit that fatality
rates in a particular year are (in part) caused by the status of
MLDA policy in that year, *not* by the change in policy. Put another
way, the highway safety outcome that one would more naturally
theorize to be sensitive to changes in MLDA policy would be
changes in fatality rates. All of Hoxie and Skinner's (1985) specifications are subject to this criticism, and thus there is reason to
question whether that study contains estimates that can be reasonably interpreted as reflecting parameters of policy interest.

The second issue of general concern raised by the Hoxie and
Skinner (1985) analysis pertains to the strategy of calculating
numerous regressions and using hypothesis testing or fitting criteria in order to arrive at a "final" or "best" specification. Such
procedures are formally described as involving "pretesting," and
informally by the pejorative terms "fishing" and "data mining."
Pretesting procedures are widely employed, but at best generate

estimates that cannot reasonably be interpreted with reference to any available statistical theory. In classical statistics, estimates can be interpreted only with reference to the sampling properties of the *procedure* (commonly called an "estimator") used to arrive at the estimates. Unfortunately, the sampling properties of all but extremely simple instances of pretest estimators are unknown; since these procedures are very complicated, it is hardly surprising that analysis of their sampling properties is intractable.

Thus the common practice of invoking standard textbook results to interpret estimates produced by pretest estimators is inappropriate: the textbook sampling properties refer to the procedure of performing a single regression—a procedure that is very different from the one actually employed and, hence, one with very different sampling properties. Even many statistics and econometrics textbooks slight this issue, apparently because of the lack of any satisfactory prescription that can be provided in response. Exceptions include Judge et al. (1985), which is rather technical, and Kennedy (1985), which provides a useful heuristic discussion.

A common objection to this line of argument is worth discussing in an effort to clarify this extremely important issue about which confusion is widespread. This common objection might be characterized as: "But if the 'best' regression had been the only regression run, then the textbook results would apply, and, after all, the *estimates* are the same as those resulting from the procedure of running only the 'best' regression." This argument, while persuasive to many, is based on a confusion about the nature of classical statistical inference: *estimates* do not have sampling properties; *estimators* (i.e., procedures) do. Hence, the answer to the common objection is: "Sampling properties derived for procedures *not employed* are not relevant." (As a practical matter, the following variant may be more helpful: "Sampling properties derived for procedures *very different from that employed* are very different from the relevant sampling properties.")

Hence a dilemma for applied researchers. In order reasonably to invoke known sampling properties—and thereby be able to appeal to statistical theory to interpret the results—one must not examine numerous specifications. But our instincts tell us that once we've performed a particular regression there is still more to be learned from the data! There seems to be no satisfactory response to this dilemma. The prescriptions suggested here are: (1) don't examine a specification without very good (*a priori*) reason to think that its results will contain valuable information; (2) describe in detail the procedure followed to arrive at the "final" specification; and (3) report the results for *all* specifications examined. With regard to Hoxie and Skinner (1985, Model I), prescriptions 2 and 3 are not met, and one is unable to address prescription 1 because there is almost no discussion of theoretical rationales.

Asch and Levy (1987a) appear to be less vulnerable to criticism with regard to the pretest issue, if only because they eschew the common strategy of deleting "insignificant" variables—lack of statistical significance does not imply that the best estimate is zero! In this regard, however, they describe briefly (fn. 14) some specifications (the number of which is unclear) for which estimates were computed but not reported. (In fairness to the authors, the absence of this information may be attributable to the fact that journal editors must typically ration space vigorously.) But, this study presents an opportunity to raise two other fundamental issues: sensitivity analysis over specifications and selective, post hoc appeal to misspecification.

Any regression specification in this area is likely to be controversial, and many will disagree concerning the "most reasonable" specification. Very valuable, then, would be specific information concerning the sensitivity of the basic results from the researcher's "preferred" specification to changes within an interesting class of specifications. (See, for example, Leamer [1978], which discusses this issue and develops new tools for sensitivity analysis over specifications.) While Asch and Levy (1987a, fn. 14) briefly claim robustness of their major results with respect to inclusion of other independent variables, their description is too vague to be of much use. This may be particularly troublesome in light of the fact that the major lesson of at least one of the studies they cite in motivation for their specification (i.e., Graham and Garber, 1984) is that the results of traffic safety regressions can be extremely sensitive to arguably appropriate specification changes.

Also, Asch and Levy (1987a) selectively invoke misspecification, in particular measurement error. Almost everybody appreciates that no data are perfect, and many know that measurement errors cause bias. Less widely appreciated is the fact that, in general, measurement error causes biases in the coefficients of even correctly measured variables. This exemplifies the principle that if *any* parameter in a regression is estimated with bias then, in general, *all* are. (Garber and Klepper [1980a, b] analyze such biases—the former focuses on measurement error and the latter addresses biases due to omitted variables and simultaneity as well.) This principle undermines the validity of a widespread habit among empiricists: *selectively* invoking measurement error (or, more generally, misspecification) to rationalize "disappointing" results.

For example, Asch and Levy (1987a, p. 186) appeal to measurement error in their drinking experience variable to rationalize the
lack of "strong" results with regard to its estimated coefficient and,
hence, the hypothesis they are apparently championing. The major
novelty of their study is the conclusion that (p. 180) "the legal
drinking age has no perceptible influence on fatalities, but inexperience in drinking is an apparent risk factor independent of age."
But, one might just as validly invoke (even the same) measurement
error to rationalize the "weak" results of Asch and Levy with
regard to the effect of MLDA. Similar comments apply to selective,
post hoc appeal to other types of misspecification. Statistics presents many two-edged swords.

A major conclusion of this paper is that the paucity of useful (or,
at least, used) theory is the major impediment to the fruitful
development of the empirical MLDA literature. In this regard, the
relatively explicit development of an empirical model and the
introduction to the MLDA literature of the concept of "drinking
sentiment" by Saffer and Grossman (1987a) are most welcome.
While one might be uneasy with the specificity of the "drinking
sentiment" concept, and the apparent difficulty of empirical implementation, such concerns should not be allowed to stifle the
development of theory in this area. Thus, Saffer and Grossman
(1987a) will represent an important contribution, even if it achieves
nothing more than spurring discussion about theoretical underpinnings of the empirical literature. "Alcohol availability," which is
mentioned frequently in the literature but underutilized, provides
another example of a simple concept with the potential to help
researchers organize their thinking, improve communication, and
crystallize much-needed discussion of theoretical matters.

Another commendable aspect of Saffer and Grossman (1987a, b)
recalls an issue raised earlier: interaction of safety policies. In
particular, Saffer and Grossman consider explicitly both beer taxes
and MLDA. It seems most likely a priori that the effect of either
policy on youthful highway deaths will depend importantly on the
status of the other policy. Thus it is disappointing that Saffer and
Grossman did not include as an independent variable the interaction of their tax and MLDA variables. Wilkinson (1987) also
considers various policies. He posits, with no explanation, a multiplicative functional form in the levels of his independent variables,
estimated as an additive form in the logarithms. This form imposes
a specific type of interaction, but the theoretical possibility that
the effectiveness of one policy depends on the status of other
policies is not explicitly addressed.

Innovations specific to Saffer and Grossman (1987b) are also welcome. These include the additional theoretical construct of "pressure to pass a 21-year-old drinking age" and the explicit development of a simultaneous-equation model. But it seems desirable to push further. For example, the rigorous development of their estimating equations provides opportunities that apparently remain to be exploited. These involve explicit attention to the extent to which the parameter restrictions implied by their model, which were not imposed in estimation, seem consistent with the data and the mean-square efficiency gains resulting from the imposition of these restrictions.

With regard to the agreement between the restrictions and the data, many would emphasize the formal "testing" of such restrictions. This author will not. Clearly, the restrictions, like all assumptions, are "incorrect." The interesting issue is whether they are *useful*—that is, yield more reliable estimates of policy impacts. More interesting than a statistical test, it seems, would be consideration of the nature and extent of discrepancies between unrestricted and restricted estimates. The objective in doing so would be development of information concerning which elements of the model are most usefully modified.

For example, consider in Saffer and Grossman (1987b) the implied proportionality of the coefficients of the variables in X_1 across the mortality rate and drinking-age equations (the factor of proportionality is θ—see their equations [4] and [5]). This proportionality follows from assuming that mortality enters the drinking-age equation through the unobserved "pressure" variable. Thus the usefulness of the "pressure" concept might be probed by considering the extent to which these proportionality restrictions are consistent with the data. For example, it appears that three consistent estimates of θ can be computed from information in columns (2) and (3) of Table II (Saffer and Grossman, 1987b, p. 412). These estimates are 6.7 (computed from the coefficients of the beer tax variable), 11.8 (from the border-age variable), and 2.0 (the income variable). The fact that these estimates are all of the same sign is encouraging. Reasonable people might disagree about whether the quantitative discrepancies are troublesome.

Method 2: Statistical Analysis with "Dummy-Variable Controls"

Cook and Tauchen (1984), DuMouchel, Williams, and Zador (1987), and others use "dummy variables" to control for other relevant determinants of highway fatalities. Cook and Tauchen (1984) provide more explanation for choice of method than is typical in the MLDA literature. They reject the strategy of attempting explicit control of other relevant determinants of highway fatalities, writing that "results from this type of analysis tend to be sensitive to specification errors" (p. 177). While this claim is indisputable, it does not address the specification errors that may compromise the reliability of estimates based on dummy-variable controls. These can be illuminated as follows.

Direct implementation of (5.2), if it were feasible, might involve regression of y on the variables contained in the vectors z and x. Assume for simplicity that the MLDA policy can be adequately represented empirically—that is, that the elements of z in (5.2) have been appropriately specified and measured. Instead of regressing y_i on z_i and x_i, consider regressing y_i on z_i and a vector of dummy variables denoted by d_i. This regression can be analyzed by the simple device of rewriting the DGP in (5.2) and adding a well-chosen zero to the right-hand side:

$$y_i = z_i'\gamma + x_i'\beta + 0'd_i + \epsilon_i \qquad (5.3)$$

where 0 denotes a vector with all elements equal to zero.

Equation (5.3) merely formalizes the idea that in the DGP adopted for purposes of analysis—that is, (5.2)—which represents a theoretical description of the process determining the highway safety outcome, the dummy variables, by definition, play no causal role. In light of (5.3), however, the "dummy-variable regression" of y_i on z_i and d_i can be viewed as implementing the regression suggested by (5.3), with the variables in x_i excluded. This way of viewing a "dummy-variable regression" is employed because it allows application of well-known results concerning "omitted-variable bias."

For simplicity, assume $E(\epsilon_i|z_i, x_i, d_i) = 0$, a key condition for the (infeasible) regression of y on z and x to be unbiased for γ and β, and for the (infeasible) regression of y on z, x, and d to be unbiased for γ, β, and 0. Consider γ_j, the jth (generic) element of γ—that is, the parameters of policy interest in (5.2)—and g_j, the estimated regression coefficient corresponding to γ_j in the dummy-variable regression—that is, the regression of y on z and d. Application of standard results on "omitted-variable bias" or "specification analysis" yields:

$$E(g_j) = \gamma_j + \Sigma_k a_{jk} \beta_k \ (j = 1,2,...J), \qquad (5.4)$$

where β_k is the kth element of β (i.e., coefficient in the DGP of the kth theoretical, but omitted, control variable) for $k = 1,2,...K$; the summation runs from $k=1$ to $k=K$ (i.e., over all of the variables in x); and a_{jk} is the coefficient of z_j (the jth element of z) in the auxiliary population regression of x_k on z and d.

Thus, (5.4) allows a precise statement of the conditions under which the use of the variables d_i as regressors rather than x_i results in unbiased estimation of the parameters of interest—that is, $E(g_j) = \gamma_j$ $j = 1,2,\ldots J$. For all practical purposes, unbiased estimation of the effects of MLDA policy requires that the auxiliary regression coefficients in (5.4) are all zero. This condition is usefully interpreted as: each of the MLDA variables (z_j's) is uncorrelated with each of the theoretical determinants in x, holding constant the other MLDA variables and the dummy variables in d. Otherwise, this method of "controlling for x" will not succeed in producing unbiased estimates of the parameters of interest.

In general, the use of dummy-variable controls will not yield unbiased estimators of the parameters of direct policy interest. The use of d as regressors could in principle yield unbiased estimates, but it could also yield estimates with the same (or, it seems, even larger!) biases as the regression of y on z alone. It is useful to consider some special cases.

Consider an extreme case in which the use of d results in the same biases as simply omitting x (and including none of the dummy variables). In particular, this would occur if the estimators of the coefficients of the variables in d in the dummy-variable regression (of y on z and d) are all unbiased for their values in (5.3), namely zero. Thus it would seem useful to test the hypothesis that in the dummy-variable regression the coefficients of all of the dummy variables are jointly zero. If this hypothesis is tenable, one might wonder whether the use of the variables in d results in estimates of γ with biases that differ from those available by merely regressing y on z alone.

Consider now a special case in which the use of d rather than x would allow unbiased estimation of γ. Unbiasedness obtains when the dummy variables jointly "explain statistically" all of the variation in each of the variables in x—more precisely, when all of the (auxiliary) regressions of an element of x on all of the variables in d have $R^2 = 1$. In this case, all of the auxiliary regression coefficients in (5.4) would equal zero: heuristically, if no variable in x has any (residual) variation given the variables in d, then the elements of x *cannot* covary with the elements of z once we condition on d (and, thus, the a_{jk} in (5.4), would all equal zero). This special case may be reasonably well approximated in Cook and Tauchen (1984), DuMouchel, Williams, and Zador (1987), and other studies employing dummy variable controls. But it seems appropriate for the analysts to provide information to help the reader make that judgment—Cook and Tauchen (1984) are commendable in this regard (see above). Moreover, it seems worthwhile for the analysts to attempt to identify and measure those elements of x for which this is feasible in order to examine empirically how much of the variation in those theoretical determinants is "explainable" (in the sense of multiple correlation) in terms of the dummy variables proposed as "controls."

A tentative, final suggestion follows from an intuitive interpretation of the "dummy-variable" strategy. Heuristically, the variables in d are included in the hope that these variables will be credited (in the regression) with the changes in y that are appropriately attributable to x, and, because x is not included in the regression, would otherwise be attributed to the MLDA variables. From this point of view, this method might be usefully thought of as attempting to introduce variables that will "insulate" the estimated coefficients of z from the biases due to omitting the variables in x. If this is the purpose of introducing the dummy variables, it seems that it would be advisable also to include measures of the variables in x to the extent possible. In that case, the variables in d would be needed to insulate the estimates of γ from the biases due to omitting only some of the theoretical determinants, a task which seems (at least superficially) less demanding.

These suggestions are offered in the spirit of attempting to learn what we can from our theories and the data, even if this is regrettably little. In general, however, the extent to which any strategy relying on dummy-variable controls succeeds (in mitigating biases if not eliminating them) depends on subtle interrelationships among the variables in z, x, and d that cannot be probed entirely satisfactorily. Consideration of issues raised here by researchers who are knowledgeable about relationships among such variables, assuming such people exist or can be created, might be very helpful in judging the extent to which any particular choice of variables d is likely to be appropriate. Informed judgments of this type would be very valuable in the evaluation of past studies and design of future ones. But fundamentally, a particular theoretical view of the variables which we would ideally wish to hold constant is required for any useful analysis of this type. Armed with a theory, it should be possible to bring additional empirical information explicitly to bear.

Method 3: Simple Paired Comparisons

A fundamental issue raised by comparison of highway safety outcomes across two situations is the appropriate choice of a comparison group. These choices are generally explained in vague terms if at all. The fundamental concern in choosing comparison groups, it seems, is the extent to which any particular choice allows the analyst to hold constant the effects of factors other than MLDA policy. This issue can be clarified with the aid of (5.2).

Consider two highway safety outcomes i and j, where i refers to the outcome expected to be sensitive to some particular change in MLDA policy under study and j refers to the comparison group. Write (5.2) for both of these outcomes:

$$y_i = z_i'\gamma + x_i'\beta_i + \epsilon_i, \text{ and} \qquad (5.5)$$

$$y_j = z_j'\gamma + x_j'\beta_j + \epsilon_j \qquad (5.6)$$

Note that (5.5) and (5.6) allow for the possibility that the effects of changes in the variables in x differ across situation i and j (i.e., $\beta_i \neq \beta_j$). This possibility seems especially important when i and j refer to two different types of fatalities, and, perhaps, different age groups. It may be much less important in interstate comparisons that involve the same types of fatalities for the same age groups.

In keeping with the focus of the "paired comparison" studies, here y_i and y_j are interpreted as *changes* in highway safety outcomes during a particular time interval in situations i and j, respectively. Accordingly, it is assumed that the variables in z and x are also changes.

First note that for comparison situation j either: (1) $z_j = 0$ in cases in which j refers to a comparison *state* that didn't change its MLDA policy; or (2) $\gamma = 0$ in cases in which j refers to a comparison *age-group* or *type of accident* assumed not to be sensitive to changes in MLDA policy. (An immediate implication is that *relative* insensitivity is not sufficient for adequate control. This suggests that the use of other types of accidents as a control group is troublesome— for example, daytime fatal accidents may not be usefully viewed as totally insensitive to MLDA policy.) When either $z_j = 0$ or $\gamma = 0$ is substituted into (5.6), we get:

$$y_j = x_j'\beta_j + \epsilon_j \qquad (5.7)$$

Equation (5.7) merely says that for the comparison group changes in y are attributable to changes in determinants other than MLDA policy, either because MLDA policy didn't change (in the case of comparison states) or because changes in MLDA policy did occur in this state but are assumed to be irrelevant to this outcome (in the case of comparison age groups or types of accidents).

Appropriate choice of comparison groups can now be addressed by subtracting (5.7) from (5.5):

$$y_i - y_j = z_i'\gamma + (x_i'\beta_i - x_j'\beta_j) + (\epsilon_i - \epsilon_j) \qquad (5.8)$$

This equation says that the difference in the changes in the highway safety outcome between the two situations is attributable to (1) the effects of changes in MLDA policy in situation i, as indicated by the term $z_i'\gamma$; (2) differences in the two situations in the changes in the other determinants of the outcome $(x_i \neq x_j)$, differences in the parameters associated with these variables $(\beta_i \neq \beta_j)$, or both, all of which are reflected in the term $(x_i'\beta_i - x_j'\beta_j)$; and (3) "random" forces—that is, $(\epsilon_i - \epsilon_j)$. Since control of the $(\epsilon_i - \epsilon_j)$ term is beyond hope, the "simple paired comparison" method of holding other determinants constant would be deemed successful if:

$$x_i'\beta_i = x_j'\beta_j \qquad (5.9)$$

Thus the paired comparison will successfully hold constant the effects of the other theoretical determinants if both the changes in these determinants and their marginal impacts are constant across i and j.

Equation (5.8) provides a basis for considering how revealing any particular paired comparison is likely to be about $z_i'\gamma$. It also provides guidance concerning how to choose comparison groups: make $(x_i'\beta_i - x_j'\beta_j)$ as small as possible. This prescription can be used to probe considerations mentioned in the literature for choosing comparison groups: geographic proximity, climate, similar *levels* of fatalities, regional trends, etc.

First, when comparing *changes* in highway safety outcomes, choice of comparison groups should consider the extent to which the determinants of these *changes* (other than changes in MLDA policy) are similar in the two situations. Since in general we would expect that changes in fatalities result from changes in the determinants of fatalities, it is doubtful that comparable *levels* of fatalities are an important criterion in comparing changes in safety outcomes. In addition, this perspective might be usefully applied to probe the relevance of geographic proximity. For example, geographic proximity might be relevant to the extent that changes in other highway safety policies (e.g., belt use laws, drunk driving and speed limit enforcement), changes in road conditions, changes in the quality of emergency medical care, changes in weather, changes in economic conditions, etc., are similar in neighboring states.

The dictim "make $(x_i'\beta_i - x_j'\beta_j)$ as small as possible" suggests an interesting, albeit discouraging, trade-off in choosing between interstate and intrastate comparisons. To the extent that differences in parameters (β's) are less pronounced across states (for the same age group and type of fatalities) than across types of accidents or age groups, interstate comparisons seem relatively attractive. On the other hand, within states differences across situations in the values of the variables in x are likely to be much smaller than across states. This poses a dilemma in choosing between interstate and intrastate comparisons.

It would be quite helpful if analysts using comparison groups (with or without statistical projections) were to address such issues directly, providing empirical evidence when possible. Fundamentally, the theoretical determinants of highway safety need to be considered carefully. Reference to such considerations as "proximity," "trends," and "initial comparability" do not get to the heart of the matter, and thus seem not to provide a satisfactory basis for choosing comparison groups or considering the validity of inferences based on them.

Method 4: Paired Comparisons Employing Statistical Projection

This method differs from the "simple paired comparisons" in that the comparisons are based on the differences between observed and (statistically) *projected* levels of the highway safety outcome. The use of projected levels rather than "before-intervention" observations seems to involve an important improvement, relating to a well-known concern.

Projections are attempts to calculate the level of a highway safety outcome in the absence of a policy intervention, and postintervention "history," and thus implicitly take into account all determinants of the postintervention outcome other than the policy intervention (and unusual postintervention events, which are addressed by use of comparison groups). Consideration of the projection aspect of this method of attempting to control for other factors can be illuminated with reference to the general DGP in (5.2), which is rewritten here with the observational subscript of "t" to emphasize the time series nature of this method:

$$y_t = z_t'\gamma + x_t'\beta + \epsilon_t. \tag{5.10}$$

According to (5.10), the time series behavior of y_t is determined by the time series behavior of z_t, x_t, and ϵ_t. The term $z_t'\gamma$, which changes abruptly at the time of the policy intervention (i.e., because of a discrete change in one or more of the elements of z_t), suggests an "interruption" of the time series for y_t, a change in highway safety that does not represent a continuation of preinter-

vention trends. Discrepancies between the observed postintervention levels of y_t and its projected levels are attributed to the policy
intervention if consideration of corresponding discrepancies for
comparison groups suggests that such attributions are warranted.

Use of comparison groups in combination with the techniques of
intervention analysis may, however, be less attractive than use of
projections alone. In principle, extrapolation by itself may succeed
in simulating the value of y_t that would have been observed in the
absence of the policy intervention—for example, the techniques
proposed by Box and Tiao (1975) do not rely on comparison groups.
If this is the case, the use of comparison groups would be, at best,
superfluous.

Considering the difficulties in choosing valid comparison groups
discussed above, it seems that the use of comparison groups may
well do more harm than good. Thus, it seems that inference should
be based on comparison groups only if "contemporaneous history"
is a clear, rather than merely a hypothetical, threat to internal
validity. Making an informed judgment in this regard would require explicit consideration of the specific nature of the threats
that one believes call for the use of comparison groups. Such
consideration requires a theoretical characterization of the process
assumed to generate the data, and additional empirical information. At the least, one might examine empirically whether the
basic policy conclusions differ substantially when the comparison
groups are alternatively used and not used. If such differences are
policy-relevant, theoretical and empirical analysis clarifying the
validity of the comparison groups seems critical.

One criterion suggested for choosing comparison states relates
to the analysis method itself. In particular, Wagenaar (1983, p. 39)
suggests that similarity of "cyclical (seasonal) patterns" is desirable
in matching states. However, since the preintervention patterns
are estimated separately for each state (and outcome measure), the
relevance of this criterion is unclear. It would seem relevant only
to the extent that similar cyclical patterns suggest similar projection *errors* (that would net out in the comparison), but no such
connection is apparent.

The attribution of differences between projected and observed
levels to the policy intervention appears problematic for another
reason. It seems reasonable only to the extent that the other factors
(represented by $x_t'\beta$) have continued their preintervention behavior after the intervention. Once again, to probe this, one must
explicitly consider what other factors determine y. If data on such
factors are available, these could be very helpful.

In fact, Wagenaar (1983) recognizes the possibility that the time series behavior of some of the determinants of y_t may be sufficiently irregular to make doubtful the appropriateness of extrapolations that ignore this complication. In this regard, he writes (p. 51):

> *In addition to controlling for long-term trends and cycles in the baseline time series, effects of specific events known to have influenced the frequency of reported crashes were also explicitly controlled in the statistical models. Such events included the fuel shortage and decreased national maximum-speed limit of early 1974 and major changes in procedures for reporting motor-vehicle crashes.*

While explicit control of these particular factors seems advisable, the question naturally arises: What other determinants of y_t were also subject to irregular movements over time during the relevant period? For example, in interpreting his results, Wagenaar (1983) repeatedly refers to economic conditions: Why are these taken into account in interpretation rather than in estimation? Such issues are not addressed. Articulation of the *principles* guiding these decisions could be very helpful.

It seems useful to view Wagenaar's use of explicit controls for some causal determinants as a compromise between a "univariate time series" approach and an approach based on explicit statistical control of other factors. As exemplified by Harvey and Durbin (1986) and the discussions, choice of statistical method for estimating the intertemporal impacts of a policy intervention is controversial. Harvey and Durbin express dissatisfaction with ARIMA modeling, emphasizing especially concerns about the paramount importance of differencing and stationarity in that approach. More fundamentally, their philosophy is succinctly presented (p. 188):

> *Our views on time series modelling are consistent with our general attitude to statistical modelling. We believe that the statistician should seek to identify the main observable features of the phenomena under study and should then attempt to incorporate in his model an explicit allowance for each of these main features.*

This author admits to having considerable sympathy for this position, for reasons addressed in the conclusion.

Looking Forward

All statistical methods involve pitfalls. Choice among methods and useful application of a method require appreciation of these pitfalls. Here I have attempted to illuminate pitfalls in the four general methods applied in the MLDA literature. This exercise seems useful for a number of reasons.

First, it has led to the development of some constructive suggestions for the implementation of each method. Second, the framework proposed here, perhaps greatly extended, should help researchers select the most appropriate methods for their particular circumstances. Third, it appears that methods two, three, and four may be popular not because they are more useful than method one, but because the pitfalls of the three former methods are less well appreciated than the pitfalls of the latter (analysis of which fills many statistics and econometrics texts). Fourth, it is suggested that the analysis provides an extended case study illustrating the cliche that data cannot be interpreted in the absence of theory. To the extent that methods two, three, and four represent largely atheoretical reactions to the (undoubted) extreme difficulty of theorizing in this area, illustration of the claim that theory is necessary to apply reliably *any* empirical method seems useful. Without explicit consideration of theory, choice among methods and interpretation of results will necessarily be based largely on "tastes" and "instincts."

Succinctly, we are faced with a choice among four clearly imperfect approaches. This suggests most strongly that substantial research attention be devoted to sensitivity analysis *across methods*. With regard to preference for a single general approach, most promising, it seems, is explicit statistical control, but not necessarily with standard regression methods. For example, measurement difficulties and the quite abstract nature of theoretical constructs such as availability, sentiment, and pressure suggest that unobservable- or latent-variable approaches such as confirmatory factor analysis, multiple-indicator-multiple-cause (MIMIC) models, or simultaneous-equation models with latent variables might be very useful. (See, for example, Goldberger and Duncan, 1973, or Aigner and Goldberger, 1977.) If it is recognized that successful application of any method requires theorizing, a major source of resistance to explicit statistical control should abate. Moreover, major arguments for this approach have yet to be made.

One argument is the diagnostic usefulness of estimates of parameters *not* of direct policy interest (i.e., the elements of β). With methods based on explicit control of other theoretically relevant factors, the parameter estimates associated with such other variables can provide very useful diagnostic information. For example, anomalous estimates of such parameters provide a warning sign of misspecification, and hence unreliable estimates of policy impacts as well. In contrast, in the cases of other approaches, the only parameters that have clear interpretations (and thus can be judged in terms of plausibility) are the parameters of direct policy interest. Accordingly, apart from implausible estimated policy impacts, estimates based on these methods can provide no apparent information concerning the extent to which the control method was successful.

Perhaps even more important are considerations related to the fact that MLDA is merely one of many potentially effective highway safety policies. It seems that theoretical perspectives and empirical information developed in studying one highway safety policy (using explicit statistical control) would often be helpful in the study and evaluation of other policies. Most fundamental in this regard is the apparent relative usefulness of (competing) theoretical perspectives on highway safety in general. Studies designed "merely" to study MLDA seem to abandon hope concerning spillovers that might enhance our ability to evaluate other policies.

Many of the issues raised in this review are sufficiently complex to warrant mathematical treatment. The MLDA literature has benefited little from the power of mathematics as a logical tool or as a communication device. The analyses offered here suggest that even a little mathematics could provide considerable improvement. The interdisciplinary character of the MLDA issue and the promise of mathematics suggest that future research might best be undertaken by multidisciplinary teams of researchers, applying together tools and perspectives rarely at the disposal of a single researcher or researchers trained in a single tradition.

References

AIGNER, D. J., and A. S. GOLDBERGER. 1973. *Latent Variables in Socio-Economic Models*. Amsterdam: North-Holland.

ASCH, PETER, and DAVID T. LEVY. 1987a. "Does the Minimum Drinking Age Affect Traffic Fatalities?" *Journal of Policy Analysis and Management* 6 (Winter):180–92.

———. 1987b. "Young Driver Fatalities: The Roles of Drinking Age and Drinking Experience." Manuscript.

BERGER, JAMES O., and THOMAS SELKE. 1987. "Testing a Point Null Hypothesis: The Irreconcilability of *P* Values and Evidence." *Journal of the American Statistical Association* 82 (March):112–22.

BOX, G. E. P., and G. M. JENKINS. 1976. *Time Series Analysis, Forecasting and Control*. San Francisco: Holden Day.

BOX, G. E. P., and G. C. TIAO. 1975. "Intervention Analysis with Applications to Economic and Environmental Problems." *Journal of the American Statistical Association* 70 (March):70–79.

CAMPBELL, D. T., and J. C. STANLEY. 1963. *Experimental and Quasi-Experimental Designs for Research*. Chicago: Rand McNally.

CASELLA, GEORGE, and ROGER L. BERGER. 1987. "Reconciling Bayesian and Frequentist Evidence in the One-Sided Testing Problem." *Journal of the American Statistical Association* 82 (March):106–11.

COLON, ISRAEL. 1984. "The Alcohol Beverage Purchase Age and Single-Vehicle Highway Fatalities." *Journal of Safety Research* 15 (Winter):159–62.

COOK, PHILIP J., and GEORGE TAUCHEN. 1984. "The Effect of Minimum Drinking Age Legislation on Youthful Auto Fatalities, 1970–1977." *Journal of Legal Studies* 13 (January):169–90.

COOK, THOMAS D., and DONALD T. CAMPBELL. 1979. *Quasi-Experimentation: Design and Analysis Issues for Field Settings*. Boston: Houghton Mifflin.

DONELSON, A. C., D. J. BEIRNESS, and D. R. MAYHEW. 1987. "The Drinking-Age Issue: A Critical Examination." The Traffic Injury Research Foundation of Canada, Ottawa, January.

DOUGLASS, RICHARD L., 1980. "The Legal Drinking Age and Traffic Casualties: A Specific Case of Changing Alcohol Availability in a Public Health Context." Chapter 6 in Henry Wechsler (ed.), *Minimum-Drinking Age Laws: An Evaluation*. Lexington, Mass.: Lexington Books.

DuMOUCHEL, WILLIAM, ALLAN F. WILLIAMS, and PAUL ZADOR. 1987. "Raising the Alcohol Purchase Age: Its Effects on Fatal Motor Vehicle Crashes in Twenty-six States." *Journal of Legal Studies* 16 (January):249–66.

FERREIRA, JOSEPH JR., and ALAN SICHERMAN. 1976. "The Impact of Massachusetts' Reduced Drinking Age on Auto Accidents." *Accident Analysis and Prevention* 8:229–39.

GARBER, STEVEN, and STEVEN KLEPPER. 1980a. "Extending the Classical Normal Errors-in-Variables Model." *Econometrica* 48 (September):1541–46.

———. 1980b. "On the Diffusion of Inconsistencies in Linear Regression." *Economics Letters* 6 (December):125–29.

General Accounting Office, (GAO). 1987. *Drinking-Age Laws: An Evaluation Synthesis of Their Impact on Highway Safety*, March.

GOLDBERGER, ARTHUR S., and OTIS DUDLEY DUNCAN (EDS.). 1973. *Structural Equation Models in the Social Sciences*. New York: Seminar Press.

GRAHAM, JOHN D., and STEVEN GARBER. 1984. "Evaluating the Effects of Automobile Safety Regulation." *Journal of Policy Analysis and Management* 3 (Winter):263–74.

HARVEY, A. C., and J. DURBIN. 1986. "The Effects of Seat Belt Legislation on British Road Casualties: A Case Study in Structural Time Series Modelling." *Journal of the Royal Statistical Society (Series A)* 147:187–227.

HINGSON, RALPH W., NORMAN SCOTCH, THOMAS MANGIONE, ALLAN MEYERS, LEONARD GLANTZ, TIMOTHY HEEREN, NAN LIN, MARC MUCATEL, and GLENN PIERCE. 1983. "Impact of Legislation Raising the Legal Drinking Age in Massachusetts from 18 to 20." *American Journal of Public Health* 73 (February):163–70.

HOSKIN, ALAN F., DON YALUNG-MATHEWS, and BARBARA A. CARRARO. 1986.

"The Effect of Raising the Legal Minimum Drinking Age on Fatal Crashes in 10 States." *Journal of Safety Research* 17 (Fall):117–21.

HOXIE, PAUL, and DAVID SKINNER. 1985. "A Statistical Analysis of the Effects of a Uniform Minimum Drinking Age." Final Report to the U.S. Department of Transportation (No. FR-45-U-NHT-86-08), November.

JUDGE, GEORGE E., W. E. GRIFFITHS, R. CARTER HILL, HELMUT LUTKEPOHL, and TSOUNG-CHAO LEE. 1985. *The Theory and Practice of Econometrics*. New York: John Wiley & Sons.

KENNEDY, PETER. 1985. *A Guide to Econometrics*, 2d ed. Cambridge, Mass.: MIT Press.

LEAMER, EDWARD E. 1978. *Specification Searches: Ad Hoc Inference with Nonexperimental Data*. New York: John Wiley & Sons.

MADDALA, G. S. 1977. *Econometrics*. New York: McGraw-Hill.

MALES, MIKE A. 1986. "The Minimum Purchase Age for Alcohol and Young-Driver Fatal Crashes: A Long-Term View." *Journal of Legal Studies* 15: (January):181–211.

MCCAIN, LESLIE J., and RICHARD MCCLEARY. 1979. "The Statistical Analysis of the Simple Interrupted Time-Series Quasi-Experiment." In Thomas D. Cook and Donald T. Campbell (eds.), *Quasi-Experimentation: Design and Analysis Issues for Field Settings*. Boston: Houghton Mifflin.

NAOR, ELLEN M., and RAYMOND D. NASHOLD. 1975. "Teenage Driver Fatalities Following Reduction in Minimum Drinking Ages." *Journal of Safety Research* 7 (June):74–79.

OAKES, MICHAEL. 1986. *Statistical Inference: A Commentary for the Social and Behavioural Sciences*. New York: John Wiley & Sons.

SAFFER, HENRY, and MICHAEL GROSSMAN. 1987a. "Beer Taxes, the Legal Drinking Age, and Youth Motor Vehicle Fatalities." *Journal of Legal Studies* 16 (June):351–74.

———. 1987b. "Drinking Age Laws and Highway Mortality Rates: Cause and Effect." *Economic Inquiry* 25 (July):403–17.

WAGENAAR, ALEXANDER C. 1982. "Preventing Highway Crashes by Raising the Legal Minimum Age for Drinking: An Empirical Confirmation." *Journal of Safety Research* 13 (Summer):57–71.

———. 1983. *Alcohol, Young Drivers, and Traffic Accidents: Effects of Minimum Age Laws*. Lexington, Mass.: Lexington Books.

———. 1986. "Preventing Highway Crashes by Raising the Legal Minimum Age for Drinking: The Michigan Experience 6 Years Later." *Journal of Safety Research* 17 (Fall):101–09

WAGENAAR, ALEXANDER C., and RICHARD G. MAYBEE. 1986. "The Legal Minimum Drinking Age in Texas: Effects of an Increase from 18 to 19." *Journal of Safety Research* 17 (Winter):165–78.

WHITEHEAD, PAUL C. 1980. "Research Strategies to Evaluate the Impact of Changes in the Legal Drinking Age." In Henry Wechsler (ed.); *Minimum-Drinking Age Laws: An Evaluation*. Lexington, Mass.: Lexington Books.

WILKINSON, JAMES T., 1987. "Reducing Drunken Driving: Which Policies Are Most Effective?" *Southern Economic Journal* 54 (October):322–34.

WILLIAMS, ALLAN F. 1986. "Comment on Males." *Journal of Legal Studies* 15 (January):213–17.

WILLIAMS, ALLAN F., PAUL L. ZADOR, SANDRA S. HARRIS, and RONALD S. KARPF. 1983. "The Effect of Raising the Legal Minimum Drinking Age on Involvement in Fatal Crashes." *Journal of Legal Studies* 12 (January):169–79.

COMMENTS BY ALEXANDER C. WAGENAAR

Garber provides a stimulating and well-written discussion on a number of methodological issues in the extant research on the effects of minimum legal drinking age policies. He correctly points out that most drinking age research has focused on the existence of a plausibly causal relationship between changes in the minimum age and the magnitude of any such effects. I think most researchers in the field are now confident that changing the legal age has a causal connection to traffic crashes among youth, and that implementing or removing legal access to alcohol for young people has an effect on specific categories of crash injuries and deaths of between 5 and 20 percent. It is useful to recall that a number of social scientists in the early 1970s argued that the higher legal ages (e.g., 21 versus 18) had no effect or even a detrimental effect on morbidity and mortality. When I began to examine the consequences of raising the age from 18 to 21 in the late 1970s, I expected a very small magnitude of effect, despite documented increases in traffic crash indicators following reductions in the legal age in the early 1970s. My rationale was that lowering the legal age significantly expanded the availability of alcohol to a major age group, encouraging the development of new drinking patterns. However, once those new patterns became habits, it would be significantly more difficult to reverse them. In short, I assumed it was easier to learn a new habit than unlearn an old one. Now that the existence of a causal link between age policy and traffic crashes is well established,[1] Garber very usefully pushes us to move on to the identification of multiple dimensions of legal age and conceptually related policies, and the evaluation of ways in which the various dimensions interact in affecting multiple outcomes of interest.

Before getting immersed in the theoretical and methodological details, it is useful to review the objectives of applied research on policy issues such as the legal minimum drinking age. The objectives are to answer at least three, and perhaps four, questions. First, *does a given policy make a difference in valued outcomes?* A difference in valued outcomes has four dimensions:

1. Does the policy increase things that are positively valued (i.e., provide benefits) such as life (by averting premature death), health (by reducing injury and suffering), and quality of life (by enhancing enjoyment of living)?
2. Conversely, does the policy decrease valued items (i.e., induce costs), such as decrease personal freedom or consume resources for policy implementation that could be used to provide other valued items.

151

3. Are levels of these valued characteristics caused at least in part by the policy? A causal link is established by ruling out plausible alternative explanations of an empirical relationship between the policy and outcomes.
4. What are the magnitudes of the effects?

Once we know the benefits and costs that are causally attributable to a policy, they can be compared, answering the second major question of applied research: *Do the positively valued outcomes outweigh the negative?* If the answer is yes, we move on to the third major question: *Are there alternative constellations of policies that provide the same or higher levels of valued benefits at lower costs?* If there are no such alternatives, the policy under examination is recommended. It may be useful to also consider a fourth question: *Which of all alternative constellations of policies with higher benefits and lower costs can be achieved, given extant structures of political, social, and economic power?* Considerations of social power, although not frequently made explicit, clearly influence the research agenda and the nature of alternative policy constellations considered.

The drinking age literature up to this point has largely focused on the first question listed above—that is, on determining whether the legal age is causally related to traffic crash involvement, and secondly, measuring the magnitude of the legal age effects. One of Garber's main points is that we need to develop much broader theories concerning (1) determinants of traffic crashes, (2) dimensions of traffic safety regulations and alcohol availability policies, and (3) how all of these concepts and variables interact in a system that produces specific sets of outcomes. To this end, we should be much more explicit about the implicit theories that guide much of our research. Development of richer and more explicit models of the interacting safety system would facilitate meeting the research objectives. Theory will (1) help identify possible effects of policies and guide the design of research and data collection efforts to measure those effects, (2) strengthen the plausibility of causal interpretations of observed relationships, and (3) help identify alternative policy constellations to meet the stated objectives of reducing injuries and deaths in the least costly manner. I completely agree with Garber that additional efforts on theory development are warranted, and are likely to provide a major contribution in meeting the research objectives outlined here. However, it's worth noting that a research objective common (at least in some degree) to all scientists was not included above—namely, achieving a complete understanding of the full system of interacting mechanisms that cause specific outcomes. For most of us, such understanding of the world is intrinsically interesting and worthwhile. However, some researchers conducting studies of the drinking age and other policies have a mission that focuses on understanding the effects of specific feasible policy options that are currently or about to be on public agenda for consideration. Their objective is not complete understanding of the entire system, but rather determination of whether a specific policy makes a difference in a valued outcome.

Garber's spur toward greater attention to theory development is a major contribution. It is when he ties theory development to specific methods that I differ. He argues that quasi-experimental research designs are atheoretical, and are used because of a lack of extant theory and to avoid the difficulty of developing and testing new theories regarding traffic safety or alcohol availability. Garber suggests that explicit statistical control (via regression methods and extensions) for all factors influencing the dependent variable under examination is the most promising way to build theory. I think his focus on statistical control of "extraneous" variance rather than (quasi) experimental design methods of control is a result of his training "as an economist and econometrician" (p. 2).[2]

Theory guides the design and implementation of quasi-experimental studies just as it guides (or should guide) *any* data analyses. We have some reason to expect that policies such as the legal age for drinking may affect traffic crashes. A simple model might be:

legal age→drinking patterns→alcohol-impaired driving→rates of alcohol-related crashes

A single quasi-experimental study may not test hypotheses concerning every link in this model, and is not likely to test hypotheses concerning all possible (exogenous) factors that affect each of the concepts in this simple model. But it is not accurate to imply, as I think Garber does, that a study is atheoretical if it does not test every possible link in the full interacting system producing the outcome of interest. The objective of most quasi-experimental studies is to determine beyond any reasonable doubt the existence and magnitude of causal relationships between some important subset of the complete causal system. This is achieved by preventing the effects of other variables in the system from corrupting estimates of effects of the focal variables. The effects of many of these other variables are controlled without requiring that the nature of the relationships be specified in advance, and without requiring measurement of each variable. A strength of quasi-experimental studies is that they establish with a high degree of confidence bivariate building blocks for more comprehensive models of traffic crashes.

The operational objective of any research study is to analyze and control variance. There are two major ways to control variance: research *design* and statistical *analyses*. Design controls involve manipulation of the level of a variable and manipulation of who experiences it. Statistical control involves examination of covariance patterns among variables. Design controls are preferable to statistical controls because of the higher levels of internal validity achieved, that is, the higher levels of confidence they provide for a causal interpretation of observed relationships. Statistical control of variance requires adequate specification in advance of a comprehensive theory for the full system of interacting factors. Experimental control of variance only requires that some portion of the full model be hypothesized and tested, while permitting control of other factors, many of which have not yet been adequately specified. Because theory in this field has not advanced to the point of consensus on the relevant variables and the nature of their interactions, any complex model proposed and tested via statistical rather than experimental controls is subject to endless debate concerning the correct specification of the model. Furthermore, some of the relevant factors influencing traffic crashes have not yet even been identified, and many factors that have been proposed are not currently measurable, and therefore cannot be controlled statistically.

An optimum study, it seems to me, would involve long time series measures of the outcome variables for a large number of groups formed by random assignment of individuals to groups from a subject pool that is a random sample of the population. Furthermore, various levels for all dimensions of the independent variables (including hypothesized interactions) would be administered to separate groups; changes in outcome variables would be compared across groups receiving the various treatments and compared with a group receiving no change in these factors. Clearly this ideal is never achieved, and most traffic safety studies using (quasi) experimental designs manipulate only one variable (or vector if we specify multiple dimensions of a concept such as "legal drinking age"). In examining natural experiments such as the legal age, the scientist does not have the power to manipulate policy to, say, try a higher legal age alone in one jurisdiction, an increase in alcohol prices (via excise taxes) in another, and simultaneous implementation of both policies in a third. Typically, effects of one policy change (or set of changes if the policy is conceptualized as a vector of dimensions) on a limited set of outcome indicators is examined in any given study. Several means are used to control variance due to unmanipulatable factors. Multiple comparison groups are examined, which are as similar as possible to the group experiencing the manipulated variable on dimensions possibly related to the outcomes of interest. Longitudinal data and interrupted time series are used to control for factors that are major differences between groups but change only very slowly over time (such as "drinking sentiment" mentioned by Garber). In a simple paired comparison design (without time series) with comparison groups differing on a dimension thought to be relevant to the outcome measured, that difference should be controlled statistically. In a time series design, if a factor thought to be relevant influenced longitudinal data at some time but not other times (within the time window under study), that factor should be controlled statistically.[3] Finally, there is another reason we may wish to control for some factors statistically in a quasi-experimental design. If we are confident that a specific factor is a major causal influence on the outcome variable under examination, statistical control of that factor may significantly increase the ability to detect small policy effects by reducing error variance (i.e., increasing statistical power).

However, we are now back to the problems of specification error that plague studies based solely on statistical control. Identification of group differences or differences over time that "may be relevant" to the outcome require prior knowledge of those factors, or in other words, require a plausible theory for their effects. Garber's point is well taken that when such statistical controls are added to a quasi-experimental design, the theory (and extant research evidence) for inclusion of each control variable should be made explicit.

In the course of discussing most appropriate methods to facilitate the development of highway safety or alcohol availability theory, Garber makes a number of excellent comments and suggestions on a variety of methodological issues. The first I wish to highlight is his point that failure to reject the null hypothesis "does not imply that the best estimate of the effect is zero" (p. 121). Some drinking age research studies have required a 20 or 25 percent effect of the policy change before achieving statistical significance, even though other studies regularly show effects in the 10 to 15 percent range, very rarely over 20 percent. Even if scientists recognize that such studies do not establish that the legal age has no effect, participants in policy debates typically use such results to argue the policy has no effect. The statistical power of a study should be sufficient to

detect the magnitude of effect our theory and previous experience
lead us to expect. All reports on policy evaluations should be
encouraged to report ex post facto power analyses, indicating the
smallest effect the study could have identified, and comparing it
with the magnitude of effect expected. If the true policy effects are
quite small, it may be impossible to design a feasible study that
can detect the effect. Nevertheless, a large number of studies all
with (nonsignificant) effect estimates that are in the same direction
might indicate policy effect that may have substantive significance.[4]
For a primitive meta-analysis, let us imagine there were 20 studies
on the effects of increasing the drinking age on traffic crashes, all
with nonsignificant results, but 18 of the 20 have negative parameter estimates. Furthermore, let us make some conventional assumptions that each study is independent from the others (policy
changes in different jurisdictions evaluated with independent
sources of data, etc.). In terms of the conventional coin toss
nomenclature of binomial theory, what is the probability that we
would expect 18 tails (negative parameter estimates) and two heads
(positive parameter estimates) out of 20 coin flips? Assuming a true
coin (null hypothesis of zero policy effect is true), a result of 18 out
of 20 tosses to be heads is expected only twice out of 10,000 tries.
With such a scenario, the best conclusion may be that the policy
reduced traffic crashes, despite all 20 studies finding "no significant
effect."

The amount of statistical power frequently interacts with measurement quality. It is generally agreed that indicators of fatal
crashes are better than indicators of nonfatal crashes. But there are
only a few fatal crashes and many more nonfatal crashes. When
evaluating the effects of state-specific policies that affect only a
limited segment of the population (like a narrow age group), there
frequently are not enough fatal crashes for adequate statistical
power. For example, in many populous states there may be only
100 fatalities per year in the category of interest, with the exact
frequency randomly jumping up and down by some 20 per year.
In other words, the natural background variation is 20 percent,
making identification of a 10 percent policy effect difficult. In such
cases, analyses of the much larger number of traffic injuries may
be recommended.[5] In some research reports the base number of
cases analyzed is obscured by presentation of rates and proportions. Graphic display of raw frequencies are recommended to
facilitate readers' interpretation of the results.

When discussing selection of comparison groups for quasi-experimental designs, Garber indicates that it is not important to have
groups with the same *level* of the outcome variable, but rather that
determinants of *changes* in the outcome are similar across groups.

I agree with this point with one qualification. It may be useful to have similar levels of statistical power across groups if changes are analyzed separately for each group, then compared across groups.

Garber suggests that "use of comparison groups in combination with the techniques of intervention analysis may . . . be less attractive than use of projections alone" (p. 144) because we do not know whether comparison groups are in fact comparable (i.e., identical on all relevant dimensions). He recommends that comparison groups be used with interrupted time-series designs only when history is a clear, rather than only hypothetical, threat to internal validity. However, the difficulty again is that we do not know a priori whether history is a problem in any given study. Use of comparison groups helps in the assessment of whether history is a threat to a causal interpretation of the observed relationship between policy and outcome. Nevertheless, most comparison groups are admittedly less than ideal. Therefore, one should analyze the intervention group by itself for a discontinuity at the time of policy change, and present results for that group alone along with similar estimates for comparisons groups, rather than presenting combined "intervention group relative to comparison group" estimates. If readers do not like the comparison groups chosen, they can examine the intervention group estimates alone. In any event, if comparison group results are consistent with hypotheses, they strengthen confidence in a causal interpretation of the observed relationship between policy and outcome in the intervention group.

Garber argues that longitudinal studies measure short-term effects and cross-sectional studies measure long-term effects. Since long-term effects are usually deemed more important than short-term (i.e., "temporary") effects, cross-sectional designs seem preferred. However, a major criterion for establishing a causal relationship is that the presumed cause demonstrably changes before the presumed effect is observed. Longitudinal designs straightforwardly establish the proper time sequence, but cross-sectional designs do not necessarily rule out the possibility of reverse causation. Longitudinal or time series designs also have other advantages. Many factors expected to have substantial effects on behavior (such as culture and social norms) vary widely from jurisdiction to jurisdiction, but change only very gradually over time. The multiple dimensions of constructs such as culture and social norms and the nature of their interactions are extremely difficult to specify. Nevertheless, such constructs can be well controlled by examining a single jurisdiction over time.

In conclusion, Garber has provided a significant addition to the policy evaluation literature. His most important contribution is encouragement of further efforts on theory development in the highway safety and alcohol studies fields. I disagree with his view that statistical control methods rather than quasi-experimental methods are best suited to facilitating theory development. We need to use quasi-experimental designs whenever possible to build confidence in causal interpretations of observed relationships, *combined with* statistical controls for factors not subject to manipulation. Combining the strengths of each method will maximize contribution to development of theory and selection of effective public policy.

Endnotes

1. Although Garber may not necessarily agree with my assessment.
2. Of course, Garber is free to point out that my perspectives are a result of my identification as an applied sociologist and public health scientist.
3. For example, evaluations of legal age policy changes typically use morbidity or mortality outcome indicators. If the same jurisdiction that changed their legal age implemented a compulsory seat belt use policy a year after the age was changed, effects of the belt use policy should be controlled statistically when estimating the effect of the age change.
4. For example, a small policy effect may be important if implementation costs are very low, and there are few alternatives.
5. Some outcome indicators are examined more than others because of the interests of external constituencies. For example, mass media reporters as well as policy makers typically want to know how many lives are saved by a policy. Number of injuries or crashes averted is less dramatic and less suited for use in policy debates, according to their perspective. Reporters and policy makers also typically want point estimates, not ranges, heightening the concern with the width of confidence bands (influenced by statistical power).

COMMENTS BY HERB M. SIMPSON

The central thesis of Professor Garber's work is that the methods used by researchers studying minimum legal drinking age laws have inherent weaknesses and have frequently been applied inappropriately, and that potentially useful research designs have been often excluded or are seriously underrepresented in the literature. It is difficult to disagree with that thesis, so, in general terms, the critique of his work is quite easy. On the other hand, this task is complicated by the fact that, unlike Professor Garber, I have not been trained as an econometrician, so I do not feel qualified to comment on the technical merits of the manuscript. This is most unfortunate, since many similarly untrained researchers may shy away from the manuscript, owing to the proliferation of formulas in some sections and, thereby, miss important messages contained in it. The paper could benefit from an incisive technical review and a more "casual" approach to formulas for the uninitiated. My critique is restricted to more general issues raised in Chapter 5.

I respect the approach Professor Garber has taken. In particular, he has offered a very constructive criticism of the methodological shortcomings in the literature. His "wrecking" exercise is well disguised—even with respect to the weaker methods, he has been constructive by suggesting how they can be improved. Perhaps this reflects more a stroke of realism than of humanity, since he recognizes that even if he shreds these methods, they will continue to be used—so, why not try to improve their application. In this respect, I believe he has made a useful contribution to the literature by softly opening methodological debate rather than guaranteeing defensive posturing.

By illustrating the methodological diversity available to researchers who are pursuing evaluation, Professor Garber has underscored the importance of interdisciplinary "teams" and approaches to problems in this field. Indeed, he calls for more frequent interdisciplinary collaboration. This plea has been a common one for years, without much visible success. It seems to me that a significant barrier to interdisciplinary work in this area is the territorial imperative surrounding certain issues and the consequent belief structure that particular problems are the domain of particular disciplines. Thus, while I sympathize with Professor Garber's point of view, I have reservations about the success of yet another call for interdisciplinary work.

Professor Garber's work highlights the importance of the main effects and interactions of a multiplicity of variables in determining changes in the dependent variable(s), as well as the difficulties inherent in disaggregating their effects. For these reasons the paper has applications beyond the analysis of minimum legal drinking age laws. Indeed, the subject of the paper serves only as case-study illustration of methodological problems that cut across virtually all the evaluation literature in road safety. Accordingly, the paper should have considerable utility for the field in general.

The need for theory, to assist in guiding methodological choice, rather than the use of "tastes and instincts," is well made and certainly consistent with the views of many in the field. However, theory development and methodological innovation have been hampered by the practical nature of the field in which the demands of the funding sources are for immediate, bottom-line answers. Practical necessity drives the field; very few scientists are afforded the luxury of time for theory development.

Professor Garber also makes an important point about the need to examine a wide range of policy options to maximize impact and minimize costs and, in particular, the need to examine these as a "package" of mutually reinforcing/complementing pieces of the puzzle. This point is particularly salient in the area of drinking-driving where, at least in the United States, there has been almost a single-minded preoccupation with drinking age laws as *the* policy.

Finally, on a very practical level I know that this paper will be of considerable interest and benefit to my colleagues Alan Donelson, Doug Beirness, and Dan Mayhew, who have recently produced an extensive review of the drinking-age issue. They will be able to draw heavily upon Professor Garber's work in revising their own manuscript.

Now, I would like to raise a few general questions and observations for possible comment and discussion.

An apparent inconsistency: Professor Garber has provided convincing evidence that the studies conducted to date have serious methodological shortcomings, which certainly compromise the validity of their findings. He also makes a strong point concerning the need to have clear and explicit linkages between data (findings) and policy recommendations. Yet, after making these points and thoroughly discrediting much of the research in the area, he concludes with the statement that ". . . MLDA is merely one of many *effective* highway safety policies" (emphasis added). This strikes me as somewhat contradictory. Given the serious reservations he has about the knowledge base, it seems inconsistent to elevate the policy to the status of effective.

Garbage in—garbage out? Given that Professor Garber is new to this field, it would have been useful to have his comments as an "outsider" on the quality of data in this area. This seems appropriate since data quality is linked to methodology. How does the quality of data in this field compare to that in other areas with which Professor Garber is more familiar? And, to what extent is the value or potential utility of the method compromised by the quality of the data?

Economic factors: Pursuant to item number 2 above, given that Professor Garber is an economist, it would have been useful to read some comments about the significance of economic variables and the extent to which they have been adequately controlled in existing studies. There is considerable evidence that economic factors, like the business cycle, have substantial impact on traffic crash rates, particularly among vulnerable groups, like the young. To what extent are the reductions in the crash rate of this group attributable not to drinking age policies, but rather to the effects of economic conditions?

On policymaking: Professor Garber makes the point that rarely are the links between data and policy made explicit in the literature on MLDA. This is important because the laws have numerous dimensions and different data are relevant to different aspects of those laws. To this end, he suggests an idealized decision problem be considered to enhance the usefulness of future studies. I agree this may have heuristic value for refining the nature of questions asked and sharpening the linkage between what is asked and what data are relevant to those questions, but in the final analysis, I question whether or not it matters. Let me amplify. I have often been impressed by the role of facts in the political process, but impressed not in the way one might think. It seems to me, as others have argued in the literature, that facts do not drive decisions—rather, the process is best described as knowledge accretion in which facts creep into the decision-matrix and are aligned in a way consistent with, or convenient to the philosophy, moral pursuation or other sensitivities of the body politic ("how will my constituents react?"). This general issue is directly linked to Garber's study. Professor Garber has rightly pointed out that the intangible effects of the drinking age laws, particularly on the cost side of the ledger (how will constituents react, decreased respect for the law, enforcement costs, etc.), are extremely difficult to quantify. But, it seems to me that these intangibles are often the key to the decision process. If I am correct that "soft" factors are important and Professor Garber is right when he suggests we really cannot measure them, then studies in this field are actually weakest where the strength, in terms of policy-relevance, is needed. I would suggest, however, that although the intangibles are difficult to measure, we should not simply relegate them to the "value judgment box," but rather first seek assistance from other disciplines that routinely measure such factors.

To summarize these interrelated points: (1) Just how influential are data in the decision process and do we know what data are weighed most heavily? (2) Will refining the linkages between data and specific policy issues enhance the impact of scientific studies? and (3) Given that the factors important to the policymaking may be intangible or difficult to measure, should we steer clear of them or look to related disciplines for methods to measure them?

Chapter 6

SOCIAL NORMS AND DRUNK DRIVING COUNTERMEASURES

by Jonathan Howland

Introduction

Over the last decade, public awareness and activism concerning drunk driving have increased markedly. Sometime in the late 1970s or early 1980s a substantial or influential portion of the public began to perceive alcohol-related traffic injuries as a social problem amenable to remedy. What accounts for this development is unclear. Surely, research documenting that alcohol—even in moderate amounts—increases the likelihood of traffic accidents contributed to the public's understanding that the problem of drunk driving was not limited to the chronic alcohol abuser. The Alcohol Safety Action Projects (ASAP) helped to establish drunk driving as a policy issue at the state and local levels. Grass-roots activism by organizations such as Mothers Against Drunk Driving (MADD) and Remove Intoxicated Drivers (RID) organized political constituencies for drunk driving laws and focused press and other media attention on the issue. The 1982 Presidential Commission on Drunk Driving gave credence to the perception of drunk driving as an important policy question and provided an agenda for action emphasizing legislation aimed at deterrence and enforcement.

Whether the 1980s are remembered as a watershed era for drunk driving prevention depends on the extent to which public awareness and concern translate into permanent institutional

163

change and new social norms about drinking and driving. Public concern over alcohol abuse has varied in intensity over time. It is possible that the current interest in drinking and driving will diminish in the foreseeable future. Nevertheless, for those concerned with traffic safety, the present level of attention presents a window of opportunity to affect change with lasting results. In this regard, the evaluator, as informant to the policymaker, plays an important role by assessing the effectiveness of social policy.

These are interesting times for public health. Research on the epidemics of cardiovascular disease, lung cancer, and AIDS have underscored the role of individual behaviors in determining health status. We have witnessed changes in health-related behaviors which 20 years ago seemed intractable. Smoking, consumption of high-cholesterol foods, and the current craze for fitness are examples. Goldman and Cook (1984) estimate that over half of the decline in heart disease mortality between 1968 and 1976 was attributable to alterations in life-style. A change in drinking and drinking and driving behaviors is also evident. We do not know whether these changes mark the beginning of a long trend. Nor can we say with certainty how attitudinal and behavioral changes affect vehicular crash rates. Nevertheless, changes are afoot and they warrant our attention.

In the discussion that follows, recent trends in drunk driving social activism, legislative countermeasures, drinking and driving behavior, and alcohol-related traffic fatalities are briefly summarized. Chapter 6 then assesses what evaluation research tells us about the effectiveness of some public policies to deter drunk driving. Finally, an attempt is made to reconcile research findings with observed trends and to suggest directions for future research.

Recent Drunk Driving Trends

Social Movement Organizations

Two important exponents of the grass-roots movement against drunk driving, RID and MADD, formed in 1978 and 1980, respectively. The growth of these organizations is notable for two reasons. First, MADD and RID have played important roles in raising public consciousness about drunk driving. Second, the expansion of these groups indicates public receptivity to hearing and taking action about the problem. Between 1978 and 1985, 424 local chapters of these groups organized at the community level. Formation of new local chapters of MADD and RID peaked during

1983, with the addition of 113 new organizations in that year alone (McCarthy, Wolfson, and Harvey, 1987). In 1984 and 1985 there were slight declines in the development of new chapters (see Figure 6–1).

Although the total membership of MADD and RID is estimated to be only 15,750 nationally, large portions of the population are exposed to the activities of these organizations. In 1985, 55 percent of the U.S. population lived in a county having a citizens' anti-drunk driving group; 67 percent of the population lived in a county from which an anti-drunk driving group recruited members; and 95 percent of the population lived in a media market in which an anti-drunk driving group was located (McCarthy, Wolfson, and Harvey, 1987).

Media Attention

The dissemination of citizens groups against drunk driving was mirrored by media attention to drinking and driving. The number of magazine and newspaper stories, as measured by analysis of selected leading publications, increased dramatically during the early 1980s. This media coverage also peaked in 1983, with subsequent declines in 1984 and 1985 (McCarthy, Wolfson, and Harvey, 1987) (see Figure 6–2).

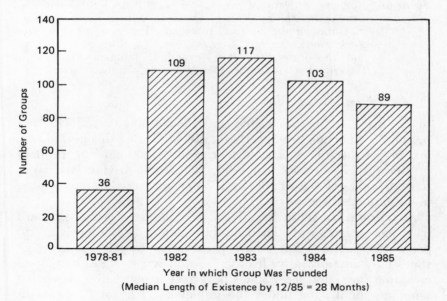

Figure 6-1   Number of Drunk Driving Groups Founded, by Year.

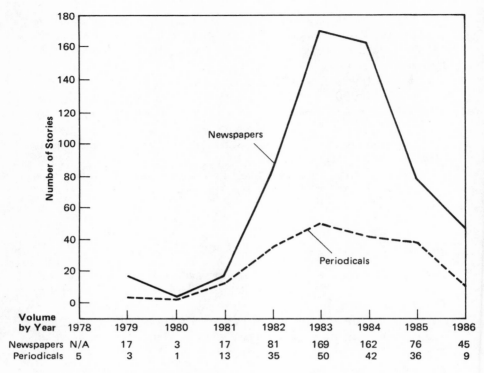

Volume by Year	1978	1979	1980	1981	1982	1983	1984	1985	1986
Newspapers	N/A	17	3	17	81	169	162	76	45
Periodicals	5	3	1	13	35	50	42	36	9

Figure 6-2 Volume of National Newspaper and Periodical Coverage of Drunk Driving, by Year. Newspaper volume based on count of stories in the National Newspaper Index; includes the *New York Times,* the *Los Angeles Times,* the *Wall Street Journal,* and the *Washington Post.* Periodical volume based on the Magazine Index. (Source: John McCarthy, Catholic University.)

Public Policy

In the five years between 1981 and 1986, states passed 729 laws pertaining to drunk driving (Hatos, 1987). During this period, the number of these laws enacted increased by 300 percent, from 44 in 1985 to 178 in 1986. In 1985, 223 drunk driving laws were passed, and as of August 1987, 1,165 new measures were proposed in 49 states (see Figure 6–3).

At present, 49 states have legal drinking ages of 21; 42 states have per se laws with blood alcohol content (BAC) levels at .10 percent or less; 36 states have preliminary breath test laws; 22 states have administrative license pickup laws; 19 states have open container laws; and most states have recent legislation increasing sanctions for driving under the influence (National Commission Against Drunk Driving, 1987).

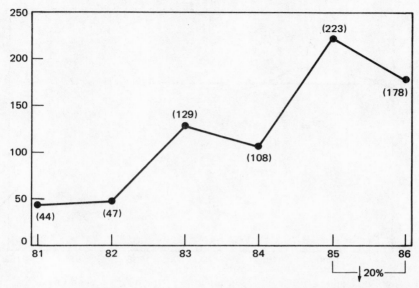

Figure 6-3 Nationwide Number of Legislative Changes to Reduce Drunk Driving, 1981-1986. (Source: S. Hatos.)

Drinking and Driving

Concurrent with the increase in public concern about drunk driving has been a decrease in reported heavy drinking and driving after heavy drinking. In 1984, per capita consumption of alcohol was 2.65 gallons, the lowest rate since 1977 (Bradley, 1987) (see Figure 6–4). Cirrhosis mortality has been declining, and in 1983 the mortality rate was the lowest since 1959 (Bradley, 1987) (see Figure 6–5). A Harris poll of a national sample of adults (N = 1,250) conducted annually since 1983 reported that the percent of drivers who say they "never drive after drinking" or "never drink at all" increased significantly ($p < .05$) from 68 percent in 1984 to 74 percent in 1986 (Taylor and Kagay, 1987) (see Figure 6–6).

Since 1984, the Centers for Disease Control (CDC) has sponsored random digit dial surveys of behavioral risk factors among adults in 15 selected states. Between 1984 and 1986 the percent of respondents who reported "driving after drinking too much" in the last month decreased in 73 percent (11/15) of these states (CDC, 1986). Overall, the mean percent dropped by 18 percent, from 5.5 percent in 1984 to 4.5 percent in 1986 (see Table 6–1). The percent of respondents who reported heavy drinking (in excess of 60 drinks per month) also decreased in 73 percent of the surveyed states (CDC, 1986). Respondents reporting heavy drink-

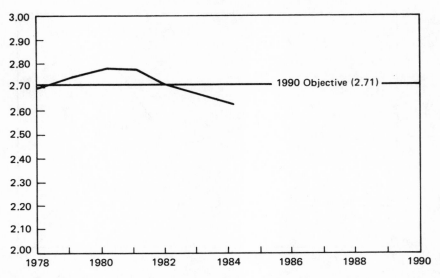

Figure 6-4   Gallons of Alcohol Consumed per Person Age 14 and Over.

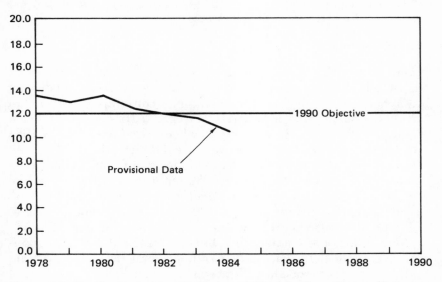

Figure 6-5   Deaths Caused by Cirrhosis and Chronic Liver Disease (Rate per 100,000 Population).

ing in the last month dropped 14 percent, from 7.7 percent in 1984 to 6.6 percent in 1986 (see Table 6–2). Binge drinking (5 + drinks on any single occasion) declined as well. Sixty-seven percent (10/15) of the surveyed states showed decreases in the percent of respondents reporting drinking binges in the last month (CDC,

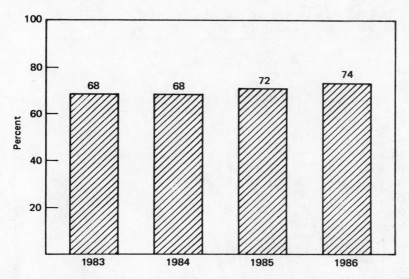

Figure 6-6   Harris Polls, 1983-1986: Drivers Who Say They Either Never
Drive after Drinking or Do Not Drive at All. Percentage point
change from 1983-1986: +6 (p = .05). (Source: Prevention
Index 1987: Year Project of *Prevention Magazine*.)

Table 6–1   "Driving after Drinking Too Much"—Centers for Disease Control
Behavioral Risk Factor Surveys of 15 States

State	1984	1985	1986	*Percent Change (1984–1986)*
Arizona	6.3	5.6	4.0	−37
California	4.2	3.3	4.8	+14
Idaho	4.2	3.3	3.6	−14
Illinois	6.9	6.3	7.3	+ 6
Indiana	4.7	3.8	4.5	− 4
Minnesota	6.9	6.8	5.6	−19
Montana	8.2	5.5	6.6	−20
No. Carolina	4.6	3.7	3.5	−24
Ohio	7.4	4.5	4.7	−36
Rhode Island	5.0	3.0	2.8	−44
South Carolina	2.0	3.3	2.6	+30
Tennessee	3.3	1.7	2.0	−39
Utah	3.9	2.5	3.4	−13
West Virginia	2.9	2.8	2.9	0
Wisconsin	11.3	9.3	9.6	−15
Mean %	5.5	4.4	4.5	−18

Source: "Behavioral Risk Factors Surveillance—Selected States," *Morbidity and Mortality
Weekly Report* 35 (16); 35 (27); 36 (16).

Table 6–2　"Heavier Drinking"—Centers for Disease Control Behavioral Risk
Factors Surveys of 15 States

State	1984	1985	1986	Percent Change (1984–1986)
Arizona	12.0	9.3	8.3	−31
California	10.5	8.2	7.8	−26
Idaho	5.8	5.9	5.7	+ 2
Illinois	10.2	10.9	8.1	−21
Indiana	8.1	4.9	7.6	− 6
Minnesota	7.7	6.6	7.6	− 1
Montana	6.9	5.9	4.6	−33
No. Carolina	6.8	4.9	5.2	−24
Ohio	8.7	7.5	9.4	+ 8
Rhode Island	8.6	6.1	7.4	+14
South Carolina	5.7	5.2	4.0	−30
Tennessee	4.8	5.0	3.7	−23
Utah	3.2	3.0	4.3	+34
West Virginia	5.7	4.6	5.2	− 9
Wisconsin	10.3	9.4	10.8	+ 5
Mean %	7.7	6.5	6.6	−14

Source: "Behavioral Risk Factor Surveillance—Selected States," *Morbidity and Mortality Weekly Report* 35 (16); 35 (27); 36 (16).

1987). The mean percent dropped by 7.6 percent from 18.5 percent in 1984 to 17.1 percent in 1986 (see Table 6–3).

Previous CDC surveys conducted on a smaller sample of states permit observation of changes in drinking and driving and binge driving behaviors over a longer period by age and sex groups. Of the 10 states surveyed between 1982 and 1985, all (10/10) showed decreases in drinking and driving among men 35 to 54 years of age ($p < .01$). Half these states (5/10) showed decreases among men 18 to 35 and $\geq$ 55 years of age, although this proportion was not statistically significant for either age group. Changes in drinking and driving among women were not significant for any of the three age groups throughout this period, but the women tended to drink and drive much less frequently than men (CDC, 1986).

A significant proportion of the 12 states (10/12) surveyed on binge drinking showed a decrease in this behavior among men 18 to 34 ($p < .05$) and 35 to 54 ($p < .01$) years of age. A majority (8/12) of states showed a decrease in binge drinking among men $\geq$ 55 years of age. A majority of states also showed decreases in binge drinking among women for each age group, and this change was significant for women 18 to 34 years of age ($p < .01$) (CDC, 1986).

Both alcohol use and use of other drugs, except cocaine, have declined among high school seniors since 1980 (Bradley, 1987). In

Table 6–3   "Binge Drinking"—Centers for Disease Control Behavioral Risk
Factor Surveys of 15 States

State	1984	1985	1986	Percent Change (1984–1986)
Arizona	20.8	19.0	16.7	−20
California	20.4	17.3	17.1	−16
Idaho	17.8	15.6	17.6	− 1
Illinois	22.8	21.2	19.6	−14
Indiana	16.6	19.3	17.7	+ 7
Minnesota	25.3	23.3	23.7	− 6
Montana	27.0	22.4	22.6	−16
No. Carolina	14.2	12.6	12.9	− 9
Ohio	22.5	19.8	20.2	+10
Rhode Island	19.2	12.9	14.7	−23
South Carolina	11.0	9.8	7.2	−35
Tennessee	8.6	6.3	9.9	+15
Utah	10.5	12.2	13.3	+27
West Virginia	11.6	13.6	13.1	+13
Wisconsin	28.9	27.3	29.6	+ 2
Mean %	18.5	16.8	17.1	−7.7

Source: "Behavioral Risk Factor Surveillance—Selected States," *Morbidity and Mortality Weekly Report* 35 (16); 35 (27); 36 (16).

1977, the proportion of 12- to 17-year olds who abstained from drinking was 69 percent; in 1982, this proportion increased to 73 percent (Casement, 1987).

Alcohol-Related Fatalities

The rate of alcohol-related vehicle fatalities remained fairly constant at 11.5 deaths per 100,000 population from 1977 to 1981; but, in 1982 the rate began to decline (Casement, 1987) (see Figure 6–7). Between 1982 and 1985, the number of drivers involved in fatal crashes increased by 3 percent, from 56,029 in 1982 to 57,844 in 1985 (DOT, 1987). But alcohol use by drivers involved in fatal accidents decreased steadily. The proportion of these drivers who were legally intoxicated (BAC ≥ 0) fell 16 percent from an estimated 30 percent in 1982 to 25 percent in 1985 (DOT, 1987). The proportion of drivers involved in fatal crashes whose blood alcohol was estimated to be between .01 to .09 percent remained relatively constant at around 9 percent (DOT, 1987) (see Figure 6–8).

There was little change overall in the percent intoxicated among nonoccupant (pedestrians and bicyclists) adults involved in fatal crashes, indicating that the decline in alcohol-related traffic fatali-

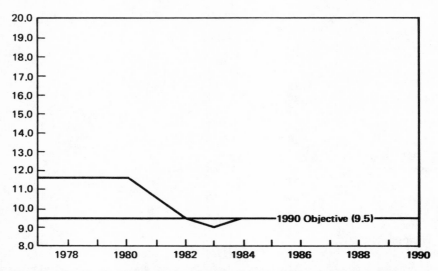

Figure 6-7 **Alcohol-Related Vehicle Fatalities (Rate per 100,000 Population).**

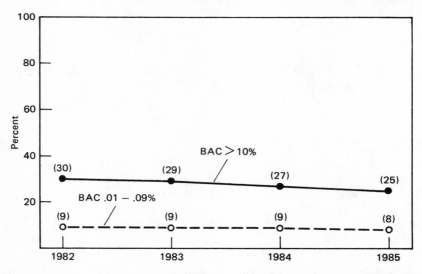

Figure 6-8   Blood Alcohol Concentrations (BAC) for All Drivers Involved in
Fatal Crashes. (Source: Fatal Accident Reporting System, 1985
Annual Report.)

ties was due primarily to changes in drunk driving deaths (DOT,
1987).

Although drivers in all age groups showed declines in alcohol-
related traffic fatalities, teenagers (16 to 19 years) showed the
greatest change. Among this age group, the proportion intoxicated

fell by 29 percent, from 29 percent in 1982 to 20 percent in 1985 (DOT, 1987).

Over the four-year period, the percent of drivers involved in fatal crashes on weekends declined 10 percent, from 38 percent in 1982 to 34 percent in 1985 (DOT, 1987). In contrast, the percent of drivers involved in fatal crashes on weekdays declined 19 percent, from 23 percent in 1982 to 19 percent in 1985 (DOT, 1987).

Similarly, the percent of drivers involved in fatal traffic accidents occurring between 6:00 P.M. and midnight, and from midnight to 6:00 A.M., fell by only 11 percent and 4 percent, respectively, from 1982 to 1985, but by much more for crashes occurring between 6:00 A.M. and noon (18 percent) and noon to 6:00 P.M. (19 percent) (DOT, 1987).

In their analysis of alcohol-related traffic fatalities between 1982 and 1984, Fell and Klein (1986) report that there was only a slight decrease (5 percent) in the percent of drivers involved in alcohol-related crashes with one or more prior DWI (driving while intoxicated) convictions who were intoxicated at the time of crash.

Summary of Trends

These trends suggest that some policies or activities concerned with drunk driving are having desired effects. Intoxication among drivers involved in fatal accidents is down, while light to moderate alcohol exposure remained relatively unchanged. This is consistent with the CDC surveys reporting decreases in driving after heavy drinking. Either (1) some heavy drinkers who drive are drinking less, while simultaneously some light to moderate drinkers who drive stopped driving after drinking, or (2) light to moderate drinkers who drive did not change their behavior, while heavy drinkers either stopped drinking or stopped driving after drinking.

The fact that alcohol-related traffic fatalities have declined among all age and sex groups indicates that these effects are generalized. The public either believes that their chance of getting caught driving drunk has increased or that driving drunk is dangerous and inappropriate.

Alcohol-related fatalities have also decreased among teens for both occupant and nonoccupant accidents. Although there were fewer teens in 1985 than in 1982, the involvement of this age group in fatal crashes did not significantly change in number. This indicates a general decrease in alcohol exposure among teens, which would be consistent with the effects of laws raising the minimum drinking age.

Single vehicle crashes are most apt to involve drunk driving. Late night crashes (between mignight and 6:00 A.M.) are most apt to involve problem drinkers. The fact that alcohol-related late night crashes have not declined appreciably, coupled with the fact that there was little decrease in alcohol involvement among drivers with prior DWI arrests, suggests that those policies which seem to affect the population as a whole may be less effective for problem drinkers.

In summary, it appears as though efforts to reduce drunk driving are having positive impacts for a broad spectrum of society. Most of the population appears to be driving less after drinking, or at least after heavy drinking. Most adults may be maintaining consumption but are separating drinking and driving either because they believe that the chance of getting caught has materially increased or that drunk driving is dangerous and inappropriate behavior. Teens are either drinking less or changing where they drink so as to avoid contact with vehicles after drinking. Problem drinkers appear to remain relatively unaffected.

Evaluation of Drunk Driving Policies

To the policymaker, recent trends in drinking and driving must be gratifying. Public concern remains high after almost a decade, people report drinking and driving after drinking less often, and alcohol-related traffic fatalities have been decreasing. Yet, however positive, these trends pose something of a puzzle to the researcher who is charged with attributing effects to specific interventions. What exactly is it that is causing these trends? And, how do we untangle the impacts of many interventions implemented simultaneously?

The question I would like to consider here is how well the results of our research explain or predict trends over time. To what extent can the results of our observations and experimentation with specific drunk driving strategies be reconciled with the apparent decrease in drinking and driving over the last five years.

Two important generic approaches to the problem of drunk driving are (1) legal sanctions intended to deter driving after drinking and (2) mass education intended to persuade the public not to drive after drinking.

From the work of Ross (1982) we have learned that the effects of deterrence laws are evanescent. The Scandinavian-type countermeasures have effects only to the extent that they alter the public's perception of the probability of apprehension. When these laws are enacted with little fanfare or debate (as in Australia and New Zealand), this impact appears negligible. When enactment is surrounded by controversy (as in Great Britain and France), effects can be dramatic but short-lived (Ross, 1982).

Ross (1982) concludes that the evanescence of deterrence and enforcement strategies is a function of the moral environment in which these interventions operate. He notes that traffic law is virtually the only important social control influence present; that traffic violations are the quintessential mala prohibita, or acts which in the absence of law will violate no other social norms (Ross, 1982). Thus, without the scaffolding of an ethos about drinking and driving, deterrence can only function through the threat of apprehension. Since this risk will always remain small within the limits of practical enforcement, deterrence is not apt to yield long-term effects on drinking and driving.

It has become almost a truism that public health education via the mass media is ineffective in changing behavior. It is argued that education about the dangers of driving and drinking can have little impact because the public is already well aware of these risks (Reed, 1981). It is further argued that mass media messages that are not consonant with the beliefs or values of an individual's immediate social environment will be disregarded (Reed, 1981). Therefore, mass education aimed at changing attitudes will not be effective in persuading people to adopt new behaviors.

There has, in fact, been little evaluation of the impact of public education on drunk driving (Jones and Jocelyn, 1978). The research that has been conducted has not been convincing. Hochleimer (1981) cites an example of an Australian education program that was intended to portray the drinking driver as "Mr. Slob" but ended producing an endearing image with whom the public identified. A quasi-experimental evaluation of a Christmas education campaign conducted in 1971 in Edmonton, Alberta, assessed effects on knowledge, drinking and driving, and attitudes toward drinking and driving laws. The program did produce a significant reduction in impaired driving in Edmonton, while a corresponding reduction in Calgary was not significant (Liban, Vingilis, Blefgen, 1985), but no evidence that the campaign reduced fatal crashes was provided (Reed, 1981). Recently, Ross (1987) evaluated the results of intense media coverage of drunk driving issues that occurred in Britain in Christmas of 1983. Although the media attention was only partially planned—much of it involved reporting news events related to drunk driving—the combined media focus on several drunk driving stories about increased enforcement and certainty of punishment was dramatic. Crash fatalities fell by 23 percent during December when media attention was most intense. But crash fatalities returned to previous levels in a matter of weeks (Ross, 1987).

In their review of mass media programs aimed at drinking and driving, Blane and Hewitt (1977) concluded that "research findings concerning the effectiveness of public education programs related to drinking and driving suggest that messages disseminated by means of mass media may affect attitudes and knowledge levels but seldom make a significant impact upon behavior." This leads Reed (1981) to question the usefulness of public education campaigns about drunk driving. Hochheimer (1981) argues that the ineffectiveness of education campaigns is a function of their design and implementation. Both, however, would seem to agree that there is little evidence to date to support the proposition that public education is effective in changing drinking and driving behavior.

Discussion

The picture that emerges from the research literature on drunk driving interventions is equivocal. Yet current trends appear more sanguine. There are several possible explanations for this disjuncture. The most obvious is that the recent trend in alcohol-related traffic fatalities is temporary; it is simply the cumulative effect of many short-term responses occurring at different times in different places. This interpretation would suggest that current trends will reverse, and alcohol-related fatality rates will revert to previous levels. The 1986 increase in alcohol-related fatality rates would support this view. A second explanation is that the triad of deterrence modes described by Ross (1982)—certainty, severity, and celerity—has only recently come into full force; that it has taken time for the requisite components of an effective deterrence strategy, such as highly visible enforcement activities (roadblocks), mandatory sentencing, and administrative pickup, to be implemented. This interpretation would suggest that deterrence can work over the long term once a certain threshold of enforcement is achieved. A third possibility is that the moral environment which surrounds the drunk driving problem is changing in response to the combined effects of grass-roots activism, media coverage and public education, and the enactments of legal sanctions themselves—that we are witnessing the emergence of a new ethos about drinking and driving similar to that which exists in the Scandinavian countries.

At this point it is not possible to know which of these interpretations will prosper. But, for several reasons, I would like to argue for consideration of the third. First, this interpretation best explains popular support for drunk driving countermeasures as demonstrated by the quantities of public legislation enacted to address the problem. Laws, at least in a democracy, rarely occur in a moral vacuum. The level of public concern about drunk driving would seem to indicate a shift in attitudes about the moral nature of driving while intoxicated. Indeed, in Massachusetts, a seat belt law was recently rescinded for being too intrusive, while sobriety checkpoints are well tolerated (Hingson and Howland, 1987). Second, this interpretation seems supported by the duration of the trends in reporting drinking, drinking and driving, and alcohol-related fatality rates. I would agree with Ross (1981) that fear of apprehension, even if intensified by increasingly visible enforcement, must inevitably be short-lived. Finally, the development of new norms about drinking and driving holds the most promise for a sustained reduction in alcohol-related fatalities. While this does not validate the interpretation that a shift in social perceptions about drinking and driving is occurring, it does argue for consideration of this interpretation.

It is possible that an unanticipated, and unmeasured effect, of legal countermeasures against drunk driving is their contribution to the development of social mores which ultimately affect behavior. For example, in Massachusetts where we evaluated the effects of new drunk driving legislation using several measures of effect, we annually surveyed a sample of adults between 1983 and 1986. One survey question asked: "How would you feel about being arrested for drunk driving?" Over a three-year period, the percent of respondents indicating that they would feel "bad" increased from 75 to 88 percent.

Andenaes (1978) has proposed that legal sanctions function in several modes to alter behavior. The deterrent effect—the effect we expect and measure—is one mode. But, laws also function to communicate social expectations and to habituate new behaviors. New laws may help to define for the individual new standards of appropriateness. Thus, deterrence may be only the first step in a process by which behavior, initially motivated by fear of apprehension, becomes internalized. In responding to changes in social norms, as opposed to fear of apprehension, the individual becomes the monitor of his own behavior and through his actions and attitudes the disseminator of moral instruction.

Evaluation of the effectiveness of public education about drunk driving has been largely ignored, perhaps because this intervention was considered "dead on arrival" after decades of negative findings in other areas of health-related behavior change. But, it seems possible that mass education may also function to disseminate and reinforce the new norms. I cannot affirm that mass education about drunk driving is effective, but I am reminded of the common wisdom that mass education about smoking was ineffective. As with drunk driving, there was a point after the surgeon general issued his 1964 report at which the vast majority of people were aware of the health risks of cigarettes. During the weeks following announcement of the report, sales of cigarettes dropped precipitously. Within a short period, however, sales rebounded. This pattern of response is not unfamiliar to evaluators of drunk driving deterrence laws. But, in the long run, large numbers of people quit smoking for good. Did the effects of continued mass media campaigns contribute to the decline in smoking? It is hard to say. But, it would seem harder to argue that mass education did not make a contribution. I doubt that many, if any, mass media antismoking campaigns have been demonstrated as effective using traditional evaluation techniques. An exception might be the Stanford three-community study, wherein mass media were combined with a total community cardiovascular intervention. Nevertheless, I suspect that smoking continues to decrease as much in response to new attitudes about the appropriateness of smoking as to the health risks of cigarettes.

The findings of evaluation research can be shaped by the model of effect which subsumes the research design. An evaluation which assumes that legal sanctions function solely by way of a utilitarian deterrence model will not measure the effects of laws on attitudes. The notion that behaviors may change incrementally and slowly over time in response to evolving social norms is anathema to the scientific methods, which requires immediate and discrete responses to discrete stimuli. The longer the period between stimulus and response, the more difficult the attribution of causality. This poses a problem for evaluation research design.

We can, however, do more to explore normative changes with respect to drinking and driving. Research evaluating specific intervention programs should include measures of attitudinal and behavioral change, along with outcomes for traffic crashes. McCarthy, Wolfson, and Harvey's (1987) study of the formation of RID and MADD chapters provides an example. The CDC's behavioral risk factor surveys should be monitored with the same interest as FARS (Fatal Accident Reporting System) data.

We need to increase our knowledge of normative change with respect to drinking and driving for two reasons. First, it may increase our knowledge about how and why trends in alcohol-related traffic crashes change. Second, we interact with the change process to the extent that our evaluations have influence on social policy. To assess interventions as ineffective in the short term when their effects may be beneficial in the long term can discourage implementation of potentially valuable policies.

In summary, I think that the current observed trends in drinking and driving reflect real and important shifts in attitudes and that in the long run these shifts may result in permanent reductions in drunk driving crashes. I cannot demonstrate that this is the case. But, I suggest that we need to know more about the processes by which new norms are engendered and associated behaviors change, and we need to adapt our evaluation designs to accommodate measurement of these processes. It is important that as researchers we do not allow the limitations of our methods to eclipse difficult to measure but potentially important effects.

References

ANDENAES, J. 1978. "The Effects of Scandinavia's Drinking-and-Driving Laws: Facts and Hypotheses." *Scandinavian Studies in Criminology* 6:35–53.

BLANE H. T., and L. E. HEWITT, 1977. "Mass Media, Public Education and Alcohol: A State-of-the-Art Review." Final report prepared for the National Institute on Alcohol Abuse and Alcoholism.

BRADLEY, A. M. 1987. "A Capsule Review of the State of the Art." *Alcohol Health and Research World* 2:4–9.

CASEMENT, M. R. 1987. "Change from a Perspective of Five Years." *Alcohol Health and Research World* 2:32–37.

Centers for Disease Control (CDC). "Behavioral Risk-Factor Surveillance—Selected States, 1984." *Morbidity and Mortality Weekly Report* 35 (16):253–54. 1986.

———. 1986b. "Behavioral Risk-Factor Surveillance in Selected States, 1975." *Morbidity and Mortality Weekly Report* 35(27):441–43.

———. 1987. "Behavioral Risk Factor Surveillance—Selected States, 1986." *Morbidity and Mortality Weekly Report* 36(16):252–54.

Department of Transportation (DOT), National Highway Traffic Safety Administration. 1987. *Fatal Accident Reporting System 1985*. Annual Report, DOT #5, 807, 071.

FELL J. C., and T. KLEIN. 1986. "The Nature of the Reduction in Alcohol in U.S. Fatal Crashes." Society of Automotive Engineers, Inc., Schenectady.

GOLDMAN L., and E. F. COOK. 1984. "The Decline in Ischemic Heart Disease Mortality Rates." *Annals of Internal Medicine* 101:825–36.

HATOS, S. 1987. Personal communication.

HINGSON R., and J. HOWLAND. 1987. "Public Perceptions of Drunk Driving

Roadblocks: Results of a Random Digit Dial Survey in Massachusetts." Unpublished manuscript.

HOCHHEIMER, J. L. 1981. "Reducing Alcohol Abuse: A Critical Review of Educational Strategies," in M. H. Moore and D. R. Gerstein, (eds.), *Alcohol and Public Policy: Beyond the Shadow of Prohibition*. Washington, D.C.: National Academy Press.

JONES, R. K., and K. B. JOSCELYN. 1978. *Alcohol and Highway Safety 1978: A Review of the State of Knowledge*, Summary Volume. Ann Arbor: University of Michigan, Highway Safety Research Institute.

LIBAN, C. B., E. VINGILIS, and H. BLEFGEN. 1985. "Drinking-Driving Countermeasure Review: The Canadian Experience." Addiction Research Foundation, Toronto.

MCCARTHY, J. D., M. WOLFSON, and D. S. HARVEY. 1987. *Chapter Survey Report of the Project on the Citizens' Movement Against Drunk Driving*. Washington, D.C.: Center for the Study of Youth Development, The Catholic University of America.

National Commission Against Drunk Driving. 1987. *Network Newsnotes*, Spring.

REED, D. S. 1981. "Reducing the Costs of Drinking and Driving." In M. H. Moore and D. R. Gerstein (eds), *Alcohol and Public Policy: Beyond the Shadow of Prohibition*. Washington, D.C.: National Academy Press.

ROSS, H. L. 1982. *Deterring the Drinking Driver: Legal Policy and Social Control*. Lexington, Mass: Lexington Books.

———. 1987. "Britain's Christmas Crusade Against Drinking and Driving." *Journal of Studies on Alcohol* 48:476–82.

TAYLOR, H., and M. KAGAY. 1987. *Prevention Index 1987: A Report Card on the Nation's Health*. Emmaus, Penn.: Rodale Press.

p 163ii
181 - 83
v. s.
9312
9213
0114

COMMENTS BY PHILIP J. COOK

Professor Howland provides some interesting descriptive material concerning the intensity of the social and political response to the drunk driving problem. The period 1982 through 1985 was extraordinary for the prominence of drunk driving as a public issue. Howland believes that this sort of attention and public action may contribute to a change in norms, whereby the proportion of the public who views drunk driving as *mala in se* will increase. The result would be to reduce the incidence of drunk driving beyond what could be accomplished through the simple deterrence effect; in the extreme case, if drunk driving were viewed as the moral equivalent of, say, rape, then many would abstain as a matter of conscience or because of the mobilization of informal social networks to discourage this behavior. I find these thoughts interesting but will offer only one comment that is directly relevant: almost by definition, there is great inertia to important social norms. No matter how vigorous, the campaign against drunk driving is not going to have much lasting effect on these norms unless it complements more fundamental changes in culture. One might ask, then, whether this campaign is part of a more general and profound evolution in public attitudes. I believe it is, but will let those who are more adept at interpreting popular culture answer this question.

Professor Howland limits his comments to just a few of the many possibilities that I would include under the rubric "drunk driving countermeasures." The remainder of this comment is devoted to listing the possibilities as I see them, with a little commentary. My list is not exhaustive, but rather is intended simply to suggest the range of possibilities. I group the "countermeasures" into four categories.

1. *Policies to reduce drinking by high-risk groups or by the general public*. In this category are included measures specific to high-risk groups, such as the minimum legal drinking age and alcoholism treatment programs, and measures to reduce per capita consumption by the general public, such as excise taxation and restrictions on commercial advertising of alcoholic beverages. Other chapters in this volume report the well-documented effectiveness of taxation and minimum age restrictions in reducing highway fatalities. The efficacy of treatment and advertising restrictions has not been so clearly established in the evaluation literature.

2. *Policies to reduce access to alcohol by people who are driving or will be driving within a few hours*. The primary policy target in this category is commercial outlets for alcoholic beverages, including everything from airlines to the neighborhood tavern. Restric-

tions can be imposed through administrative rules (no beer served at ball games after the sixth inning) or induced through incentive schemes (dram shop liability, licensing procedures) that encourage servers to take due care in whom they serve. There is also a long list of other regulations governing the operation of on-premise servers (special taxes, opening and closing hours, prohibition on happy hours, etc.) that may have some effect on the prevalence of drunk driving where they are enforced. While the measures in this category are certainly plausible weapons in the battle against drunk driving, their effectiveness has not been clearly demonstrated in empirical work.

3. *Policies to persuade or help people to separate drinking and driving.* One general approach here derives from the assumption that many people wish to avoid driving while drunk but need to be educated about *how* to avoid it. Public messages that provide information on how much is "too much," or that suggest techniques for avoiding "too much" (e.g., have a designated driver in the group, make the one for the road coffee), are motivated by this assumption. Another approach derives from the assumption that people do not understand the dangers of drunk driving and would abstain if they were properly educated in this regard: thus people convicted of DUI (driving under the influence) are sometimes required to attend classes that teach (among other things) the risks associated with drunk driving, and public interest advertising often emphasizes the likelihood of an accident when a drunk is behind the wheel. Such educational strategies appear ineffective in empirical evaluation studies.

A third approach is to encourage would-be drivers to find another means of transportation when they have been drinking. Bartenders may call a cab for inebriated patrons, for instance. A "high-tech" measure is the experimental ignition interlock systems that attempt through one means or another to discourage drunks from starting the vehicle.

4. *Policies to deter people from driving when drunk.* The possibilities here include a wide range of measures designed to increase the perceived likelihood and severity of punishment for driving while intoxicated. Included here are new laws to increase criminal or administrative penalties, to make conviction easier (e.g., through *per se* laws), or to increase the probability of arrest by instituting road blocks, targeted police patrol programs, and so forth. Such programs are potentially effective but difficult to sustain given all the other demands on the criminal justice system.

The list of "drunk driving countermeasures" is thus long and diverse. It is wise to remember that imposing any of these measures has costs, and the benefits for some of these measures are probably negligible. Even in a political climate where the public is demanding that something be done, it is important for policymakers to recall that reducing drunk driving, while important, does compete with other valid public objectives. Given the problems of empirical evaluation work (some of which are mentioned by Professor Howland), there will always be considerable uncertainty about whether a particular action will reduce drunk driving, and, if so, whether this benefit is greater in some sense than the cost of taking this action. It is up to us, as evaluation experts, to work toward reducing this uncertainty while remaining honest about the extent of our ignorance.

COMMENTS BY H. LAURENCE ROSS

Dr. Howland's paper is based on the understanding that drunk driving has declined during the last decade in the United States. He proposed that the cause of this decline may be not so much simple deterrence as the long-range effect of a social movement and its political product that declare drunk driving to be a social menace. Following Andenaes, Dr. Howland proposes that American attitudes and behavior related to drinking and driving may be changing in the direction of those prevailing in Scandinavia, and he suggests that this can lead to fewer crash-related deaths and injuries. My reservations about this thesis begin with the fact that I am not convinced that drunk driving has importantly declined in the United States nor that the explanation for any decline need go much further than to cite changes in the economy or demography of the country. Moreover, if there is a shift in attitudes concerning drunk driving in the United States in the direction of a Scandinavian model, I doubt that this will lead to Scandinavian results in the absence of other Scandinavian conditions, such as limiting access to alcohol and providing alternatives to private automobile transportation. Finally, I don't think that Dr. Howland's optimistic evaluation of what I might call the MADD era in America pays sufficient attention to its costs.

My first concern relates to whether drunk driving has declined in the United States. Dr. Howland cites survey data to show both that attitudes and reported behavior have changed over time. However, such survey data are notoriously unreliable in cases where social desirability can affect the answers. An alternative explanation for the changes noted by Dr. Howland is that the political hue and cry of the past decade have made it more imperative to denounce drunk driving and less acceptable to admit it. For instance, I find incredible the Harris data to the effect that three-fourths of all drivers claim that they do not drive after (any) drinking.

A better index on which Dr. Howland relies is the proportion of alcohol-involved crash deaths, as measured by the FARS program. Indeed, the evidence through 1985 is as cited by Dr. Howland. However, there appears to have been an important reversal in the 1986 data, which militates against the assumption of a continuing trend for the better in these figures.

If, for the sake of argument, one accepts that some improvement in the drunk driving situation occurred through 1985, Dr. Howland's explanation is not the only one possible. James Fell, the official in charge of the FARS program, has analyzed his own data and concluded that an important part of the reduction may be due to changing demographic and economic factors. Discretionary driving is reduced in periods of high unemployment, and drunk driving bulks larger in this category than in activities like commuting to and from work. Moreover, there has been a decline in the age groups most likely to be drinking heavily. If this is not the whole explanation for the observed decline in drunk driving, an additional part may be the temporary effect of simple deterrence-based laws, and the increased drunk driving in 1986 may signal the eventual disappearance of the deterrent effect—a phenomenon that Dr. Howland and I agree has frequently been confirmed in past experience.

Are American attitudes approaching those of Scandinavians, as suggested by Dr. Howland? My first five-month experience as a Fulbright lecturer in Finland has convinced me that Scandinavian attitudes are fundamentally different from the American ones in the matter of alcohol issues, and that it is likely that the characteristic Scandinavian laws are as much a product of these attitudes as vice versa. An important difference between Americans and Scandinavians is the view of the latter that alcohol is a dangerous drug. Its proper use is to get drunk. If drunken comportment is not admired, it is nonetheless expected. Another way of putting this is that Scandinavians view man's weakness in the face of alcohol the way that Italians view man's weakness in the face of women. This is fundamentally different from the American view of alcohol, which sees it as a social lubricant and intoxication as abusive, much less the French view that alcohol is a food.

Moreover, Scandinavians understand the institutional causes of drunk driving and are willing to accept inconvenient limitations on access to alcohol and expensive subsidies to systems of transport other than the private automobile as central social policy. In my view, the American opposition to drunk driving is superficial and hypocritical. To take a national example, the President's Commission on Drunk Driving refused to recommend even a five-cent-per-drink tax in order to reduce alcohol consumption and pay the costs of other countermeasures. To take a local example, when the Niagara Frontier Chapter of RID proposed that Erie County, New York (Buffalo), align its closing hours with all other adjacent counties and Ontario in order to prevent the mass migration of drinkers being observed at 2 A.M. each night (returning even more soused at 4 A.M. when the Erie County bars closed), the County Commission fled in retreat as over a thousand bar owners, personnel, and patrons flooded the hearing room. (I am convinced that the devil himself would be welcomed in Erie County if he promised to hire a thousand ex-steel-plant workers.)

Finally, I would hope that an evaluation of drunk driving countermeasures would weigh their costs along with any benefits that may be experienced. Surely, the increasing punitiveness of American law is an important cost that we experience in the effort to deter drunk driving. The exposure of masses of generally conformist people to undignified and even violent treatment by police, financially crippling fines, and confinement in sometimes horrendous institutions is costly, as is the cognizance that we live in a society that believes these things to be proper. These policies should be recognized as deriving from and supporting the Reaganite view that social problems are a matter of individual responsibility and that individuals are morally, even criminally, accountable for their own victimization. The fact that those punished are a tiny, arbitrarily selected, minority of offenders magnifies the costs, in my opinion.

Another way in which we pay for any reduction that we may achieve from deterring drunk driving is the abandonment of traditional civil liberties. Graham Hughes has suggested a convincing parallel between police "safety check-points" and the use of dogs to sniff passers-by for drugs, or patting down pedestrians for possible concealed weapons.

The reimposition of Prohibition on a politically defenseless part of the adult population is arguably another cost we incur for possible reductions in drunk driving. If restrictions on access to alcohol are worthwhile accepting as a price of increased highway safety, their imposition on the youthful minority cannot be completely justified except in terms of expedience.

Most importantly, I feel that any gains that may have been achieved in recent years as a result of deterrence-based policy have involved the cost of distracting attention and policy from the fundamental cause of drunk driving, which lies in the patterns of transportation and recreation that characterize American society. The MADD era has given the government, the automobile industry, and the alcoholic beverage industry free passes in the matter of responsibility for the problem of death and injury on the highway. Alcohol is easily and cheaply available in the United States, now after six years of the MADD movement almost as before, and nothing has been done to offer citizens reasonable alternatives to the private automobile for commuting, shopping, loving, and drinking. The move toward requiring occupant protection—far more likely to reduce deaths than even totally eliminating drunk driving—has received little active support from the movement. In my opinion, the reasons for this lie in the retributive and vengeful motivations of the citizen activists—motivations that are understandable but seldom understood by those who are moved by them.

In brief, I would hope that Dr. Howland will complete his evaluation of drunk driving countermeasures, not only reassessing the benefits in light of recent developments in the figures on alcohol-related deaths, but acknowledging the need for entries on the cost side of the ledger as well.

COMMENTS BY ROBERT B. VOAS

Jon Howland has provided a good description of the changes in alcohol consumption and in alcohol-related highway deaths and injuries during the first half of this decade. As he notes, there appears to be evidence of a reduction in alcohol-related traffic crashes, but whether this reduction is permanent or will prove to be transitory remains to be determined. Several issues arise in evaluating the evidence summarized by Jon Howland. First, we need to evaluate the quality of the data presented. Then we must ask whether we can conclude that the data demonstrate a true change or whether they are only chance variations of longer-term trends. Finally, we must determine whether these changes, if statistically significant, can be attributed to highway safety programs.

With respect to the data presented, Phil Cook, in his response to Jon's work, has challenged the usefulness of the survey questionnaire information and expressed doubt over the reliability of the data from the Fatal Accident Reporting System (FARS). I share some of Cook's concern with questionnaire data since it is so difficult to relate this verbal behavior to the driving behavior and the official record data with which we normally evaluate traffic safety programs. Nevertheless, survey data can provide a measure of trends, providing the survey procedures and questions remain constant.

I am considerably more confident of the validity and reliability of the FARS data than is Cook. This system is, after all, an official census, which is a 98 percent complete listing of all fatal crashes. If there is uncertainty, it relates to determining the role of alcohol in these crashes. However, most states now report reasonably complete alcohol concentration (AC) data on fatally injured drivers, and methods have been developed for the imputation of alcohol involvement to drivers involved in fatal accidents for whom no chemical test results are available (Klein, 1986).

One opportunity that Jon Howland seems to have missed is a more in-depth analysis using the FARS. An example of the light that such analysis might throw on the reasons for the reduction in accidents which he reports is shown in Tables 6–A–1 and 6–A–2. Table 6–A–1 indicates the reduction in involved persons with AC

Table 6–A–1 Reduction in Alcohol-Related Crashes by Class of Road User (1982–1985): Persons with ACs at or Above .10

All drivers:	16% reduction
All pedestrians:	1% reduction

Source: Fatal Accident Reporting System, 1986, National Highway Traffic Safety Administration, 400 7th St. S.W., Washington, D.C. 20590.

188

Table 6–A–2   Reduction in Alcohol-Related Crashes by Class of Road User
(1982–1985): Persons in Fatal Crashes with ACs at or Above .10

Drivers age 25–34	8% reduction
Drivers age 16–20	32% reduction
Pedestrian age 14–19	27% reduction

Source: Fatal Accident Reporting System, 1986, National Highway Traffic Safety Administration, 400 7th St. S.W., Washington, D.C. 20590.

equal to or greater than .10. The number of such drivers in fatal accidents was reduced by 16 percent between 1982 and 1985, while the number of pedestrians at these high ACs was reduced only 1 percent, suggesting that whatever produced the change it was not a variation in overall alcohol consumption but, rather, something more specifically related to driving.

Table 6–A–2 shows another set of data taken from the FARS, which indicate that between 1982 and 1985 the number of high AC drivers in fatal crashes between the ages of 25 and 34 decreased by 8 percent, while the number of drivers under age 21 with high ACs decreased by 32 percent. Moreover, in this teenage category, the number of pedestrians in fatal accidents with AC at or over .10 decreased by 27 percent. Clearly, here are data suggesting that the age 21 drinking laws may have had a significant effect on alcohol-related fatalities. Obviously, much more is needed than these simple comparisons to prove cause and effect with respect to the alcohol-related fatalities; however, these examples illustrate the opportunities provided by the improved recording of fatal accidents.

Simply increasing the detail with which the descriptive data are presented does not, of course, demonstrate causal relationships. To persuade ourselves that an observed change has resulted from highway safety programs, we must rely on a good experimental design and appropriate use of inferential statistics. Achieving this for the broad national statistics reported by Jon Howland is certainly difficult and may be unsatisfactory at best. However, he does not apply statistical tests to the trend changes he reports to demonstrate that, in fact, a significant change has occurred. Phil Cook notes, for example, that the trend in deaths due to cirrhosis and chronic liver disease has been falling for years. The downward trend reported by Jon Howland for the first half of this decade may simply be a continuation of that longer-term trend and may have no relationship to recent changes in public attitudes toward drinking and drunken driving.

There is also a need for any analysis of this problem to eliminate "competing hypotheses." Among these are the following:

1. *Changes in the economy* (fatalities rise when the employment level rises).
2. *Demographic changes* (there are fewer teenagers as the baby boom generation ages).
3. *Changes in health attitudes and practices* (Jon Howland mentions the increased public concern with nutrition and exercise).
4. *Changes in the enforcement of national speed limits* (the effect of the 55 MPH law was wearing off during the period Jon Howland covered).
5. *Changes in state safety belt legislation and enforcement* (earlier chapters point to significant lifesavings due to safety belt usage laws).
6. *Changes due to age 21 drinking laws* (while passed as part of the highway safety effort, these laws are only indirectly related to drunken driving behavior).

We should also keep in mind that these broad national changes may not be very useful in evaluating particular pieces of legislation. Ross (1975) reviewed the changes in highway accidents associated with major pieces of drinking driving legislation in Scandinavia and was not able to demonstrate a significant relationship using time series analysis. On the other hand, Snortum (1984) and Snortum, Hauge, and Berger (1986) have found considerable evidence for strong deterrence to drinking and driving in Scandinavia when accident statistics and survey data are compared with the United States and other industrialized nations. It is probable that time series experimental designs such as those described by Steve Garber are most effective in more circumscribed studies where more of the relevant factors that influence accident rates can be controlled than in studies of slow cultural changes where a multitude of factors may enter into the trends observed.

Turning to the issue of specific countermeasure programs which may have contributed to the overall national result, a number of studies demonstrate the effectiveness of specific law changes or safety programs within a given jurisdiction over a limited time period. Jon Howland did not attempt to review these studies, perhaps because time would have permitted only the most cursory review. It is not clear, in any case, whether the national result is the sum of such efforts, documented and undocumented, or whether a larger national trend accounts for the reduction in alcohol-related fatalities. Without attempting to review this literature, it is worth noting that among the countermeasures found to be effective within these limited contexts are increased drunk driving enforcement, more severe sanctions such as longer license suspension and short-term jail sentences, and long-term treatment programs for problem drinkers (Voas, 1986). These are the types of programs which account for most of the increase in drunken driving legislation reported by Howland.

Turning to the more general issue of our progress in combating drunken driving, let me venture to suggest that really significant reductions in drunken driving are not likely until the risk of apprehension and the corresponding general deterrence to driving while impaired is substantially increased. Table 6–A–3 presents an estimate of the number of miles driven at an AC of .10 for each accident and for each drunk driving arrest in this country. On average, a driver has to make a round trip across this nation while over .10 in order to be arrested for impaired driving! Obviously, we must find a way to increase the perception of the probability of an arrest if we hope to deter the drinking driver. Innovative enforcement methods making use of "sobriety checkpoints" and "passive sensors" (Jones and Lund, 1986) may provide a method for increasing deterrence, but this remains to be conclusively demonstrated.

Specific enforcement programs have shown temporary and local impact in a number of areas in the United States (Voas and Hause, 1987; Voas, Rhodenizer, and Lynn, 1985; Lacy et al., 1986) and abroad (Ross, 1984; Homel, 1986). Despite this increased attention to enforcement, in the opinion of this writer, we have yet to try in the United States the potentially most effective enforcement sys-

Table 6–A–3   Estimates of the Miles Driven for Each Alcohol-Related Accident and Drunk Driving Arrest

---

1. Approximate annual vehicle miles of travel in the U.S. = 2 trillion.
2. Approximate proportion of miles driven at .10 AC or greater = 0.5 percent. Approximate annual miles at .10 AC = .005 × 2 trillion = 10 billion.
3. Approximate annual number of fatal crashes involving a driver at AC .10 or greater = 17 thousand.
4. Approximate annual number of drunken driving arrests = 2 million.

Therefore:
5. Miles driven at .10 AC per alcohol-related fatal accident = 600 thousand.
6. Miles driven at .10 AC per drunk driving arrest = 5 thousand.

Note: These figures are obviously most sensitive to the estimate in statement 2. The number of high AC drivers on the roads varies with the time of day, day of week, and location. At some times and places, as high as 10 percent of the drivers have been found to be at .10 AC. The 0.5 percent estimate was selected as more correct for the average for all times and places, based on a study by Fox and Borkenstein (1975) who found 1.2 percent of drivers at or above .10 in their survey of random locations, seven days a week from 7 P.M. to 3 A.M.

tem available—the system I have characterized elsewhere as "chemistry-based" enforcement (Voas, 1982a; Voas, 1982b).

Perhaps the most intensive enforcement effort implemented to date is the one currently underway in New South Wales, Australia (Homel, 1986). This program, introduced in December 1982, calls for law enforcement officers to spend a significant portion of each tour of duty in conducting random sobriety checkpoints—stopping motorists and testing every driver examined. Under this program, the number of breath tests administered increased by a factor of 8. In the first 12 months of the operation, over 900,000 BAC tests were administered, or nearly one for every three licensed drivers in New South Wales. Homel reported that the monthly fatalities were lower by an average of 23 percent compared with the previous six years during the first year of this program.

The New South Wales program illustrates what I have attempted to classify as a "chemistry-based" in contrast to the traditional "behavioral-based" enforcement system. Larry Ross (1984) has popularized the term "Scandinavian model" for those enforcement efforts that are based on the illegal per se definition of the drunk driving offense (equating the offense with a prohibited BAC), and on the use of portable breath-testing devices at the roadside. This type of system is now in place most everywhere in the United States. The additional feature encompassed by my definition of chemistry-based enforcement is the use of checkpoints to produce random testing.

The traditional *behavioral-based* approach to enforcement in the United States involves the selection of vehicles from the traffic flow based on aberrant or illegal behavior. Once stopped, drivers are interrogated by the police officer in an attempt to determine from appearance and behavior whether there is sufficient evidence of drinking and alcohol impairment to warrant an arrest and a breath test. Thus, right down to the point of arrest, emphasis is placed upon driver behavior and appearance.

In the *chemistry-based* approach as demonstrated in New South Wales, drivers are stopped at random so that behavior plays no role in the selection of vehicles from the traffic flow. Further, once stopped, all drivers, without exception, are tested. Thus behavior does not enter into the arrest process, and the enforcement system can be categorized as chemistry-based in contrast to the traditional behavior-based system.

The typical Scandinavian system now commonly used in most industrialized nations has employed some features of both systems. In the United States, for example, most sobriety checkpoints or road blocks stop drivers at random because the courts have required that individual officer discretion not be exercised in the selection of vehicles to be stopped. However, once stopped, the officers must proceed by using interviews and observations to determine which individual to arrest and test for alcohol. When this system was tried in Charlottesville, Virginia (Voas et al., 1985; Jones and Lund, 1986), we found that only 48 percent of the individuals above the legal limit who were passing through the road block were apprehended. Similarly low probabilities of detection have been found in other sobriety checkpoint operations (Vingilis, Adlaf, and Chung, 1982).

In the United States the systematic testing of all drivers stopped at random has been inhibited by a question as to whether drivers stopped at checkpoints can be required to take a breath test under the limitations imposed by the Fourth Amendment. Based on relevant federal and Supreme Court decisions, the issue seems to turn on the extent of intrusion produced by the breath test, relative to the need of the state to protect the public from drunken drivers. Court decisions have clearly indicated that a breath test is a "search," but whether the intrusiveness of that search is sufficiently great to be "unwarranted" in view of the need of the state to protect the public from drunken drivers has never clearly been judicated. In any case, advancing technology has provided police officers with "passive" sensors (Voas, 1983; Jones and Lund, 1986) which do not require the cooperation of the driver in providing a breath sample but can detect alcohol from in front of the driver's face. There seems to be little doubt that this device does not involve a "search" as defined by the Fourth Amendment. Therefore, it is not limited by the U.S. Constitution. Thus the capability exists today to carry out this full "chemistry-based" enforcement system in which drivers are stopped at random and every one stopped is examined with an electrochemical sensor for alcohol.

The checkpoint system has been criticized by some law enforcement agencies as being inefficient, since many vehicles are stopped and many drivers are examined but few are arrested for DUI. Some jurisdictions, however, are successful in making more arrests per police officer man-hour at checkpoints than in the traditional enforcement system. This was true in the Charlottesville checkpoint operation (Voas, Rhodenizer, and Lynn, 1985) in which I was involved. Using passive sensor devices it is possible to determine whether the driver has been drinking within 15 seconds. This allows those who have not been drinking to be excused almost immediately (helping to meet the requirements of the courts for minimal intrusion on the public at a checkpoint). Only those who have been drinking heavily enough to provide a threshold indication on the passive sensor are detained for further, more careful checking and a quantitative breath test. Checkpoints, efficiently run using this system, will most probably produce at least the same number of arrests per police officer man-hour as the traditional system. More importantly, they have the potential for being considerably more effective because they not only impact on those who are over the limit, but also act as a warning to all potential drinking drivers. For the nondrinker, checkpoints confirm that enforcement is active and thereby support their efforts to intervene with friends who are drinking.

It is probably not possible to determine the extent to which DUI enforcement has contributed to the significant reduction in drinking and driving accidents during the first half of this decade. However, it is clear that behavioral change must be motivated. Enforcement provides a significant opportunity to motivate safe behavior. Prior to this decade most public information programs on drinking and driving were judged to be ineffective—perhaps because they were so frequently implemented alone without any supporting change in the driving environment. Wilde et al. (1971) reviewed the public information and education (PI &E) programs in highway safety and noted that to be effective, they had to exist in combination with enforcement or other official actions.

Snortum and Berger (1987) have reported on a survey of drivers in which they note that those most at risk for DUI arrest were best informed on DUI laws. Chemistry-based enforcement is designed to convince those most exposed to alcohol-related crashes that they are at risk of being arrested—not necessarily actually to arrest them. Experience has shown that, however tragic, accidents occur too infrequently to effectively motivate behavior. As evidenced in Table 6–A–3, we are unlikely to be able to increase arrests enough to increase significantly the true probability of apprehension to the point of deterring the majority of imparied drivers.

The use of the chemistry-based system at a sufficient scale can provide sufficient visibility for the enforcement effort to create the appearance of a high probability of apprehension. Since it is the perceived probability of apprehension rather than the actual probability that is believed to produce deterrence, chemistry-based enforcement can provide the basis for supporting public education programs directed at the intervention of "significant others" with drivers at risk. Strong DUI enforcement can provide the environment in which these messages would be much more likely to be effective and, over the long run, much more likely to change basic public attitudes regarding drinking and driving.

References

Fatal Accident Reporting System (FARS). 1986. National Highway Traffic Safety Administration, 400 7th St. S.W., Washington, D.C. 20590.

Fox, B.H., and R. F. BORKENSTEIN. 1975. "Patterns of Blood Alcohol Concentrations." In S. Israelstam and S. Lambert, (eds.), *Alcohol, Drugs, and Traffic Safety*. Toronto, Canada: Addiction Research Foundation of Ontario, pp. 51–67.

HOMEL, R. 1986. *Policing the Drinking Driver: Random Breath Testing and the Process of Deterrence*. Sydney, Australia: Federal Office of Road Safety.

JONES, I. S., and A. K. LUND. 1986. "Detection of Alcohol-Impaired Drivers Using Passive Alcohol Sensor." *Journal of Police Science and Administration* 14, no. 2:153–60.

KLEIN, T. 1986. *A Method for Estimating Posterior BAC Distributions for Persons Involved in Fatal Traffic Accidents*. National Highway Traffic Administration, 400 7th St. S.W., Washington, D.C. 20590.

LACY, J. H., J. R. STEWARD, L. M. MARCHETTI, C. L. POPKIN, P. V. MURPHY, R. E. LUCKE, and R. K. JONES. 1986. *Enforcement and Public Information Strategies for DWI General Deterrence: Arrest Drunk Driving—The Clearwater and Largo, Florida Experience*. NHISA Report No. DOT HS 807066, National Technical Information Service, Springfield, Va 22161.

ROSS, H. L. 1975. "The Scandinavian Myth: The Effectiveness of Drinking-and-Driving Legislation in Sweden and Norway." *Journal of Legal Studies* 4:285–310.

———. 1984. *Deterring the Drinking Driver: Legal Policy and Social Control*. Lexington, Mass.: D. C. Heath.

SNORTUM, J. R. 1984. "Alcohol Impaired Driving in Norway and Sweden: Another Look at 'the Scandinavian Myth.' " *Law and Policy* 6, no. 1:5–37.

SNORTUM, JOHN R., and DALE E. BERGER. 1987. *Technical Knowledge of the Drunk Driving Laws as a Function of the "Need to Know."* Presented at the Law and Society annual meeting, Washington, D.C.

SNORTUM, J. R., R. HAUGE, and D. E. BERGER. 1986. "Deterring Alcohol-Impaired Driving: A Comparative Analysis of Compliance in Norway and the United States." *Justice Quarterly* 3, no. 2:139–65.

VINGILIS, E., E. M. ADLAF, and L. CHUNG. 1982. "Comparison of Age and Sex Characteristics of Police-Suspected Impaired Drivers and Roadside-Surveyed Impaired Drivers." *Accident Analysis and Prevention* 14:425–30.

VOAS, R. B. 1982a. *Drinking and Driving: Scandinavian Laws, Tough Penalties, and United States Alternatives*. Technical Report, DTNH-22-82-P-05079. National Highway Traffic Safety Administration, 400 7th St. S.W., Washington, D.C., 20590.

———. 1982b. "Selective Enforcement during Prime-Time Drinking-Driving Hours: A Proposal for Increasing Deterrence without Increasing Enforcement Costs." *Abstracts and Reviews in Alcohol and Driving* 3, nos. 10–12:3–14.

———. 1983. "Laboratory and Field Tests of a Passive Alcohol Sensing System." *Abstracts and Reviews in Alcohol and Driving* 4, no. 3:3–12.

———. 1986. "Special Preventive Measures." Paper presented at the 10th

International Conference on Alcohol, Drugs and Traffic Safety, Amsterdam, The Netherlands.

VOAS, R. B., and J. M. HAUSE. 1987. "Deterring the Drinking Driver: The Stockton Experience." *Accident Analysis and Prevention* 19, no. 2:81–90.

VOAS, R. B., A. E. RHODENIZER, JR., and C. LYNN. 1985. *Evaluation of the Charlottesville Checkpoint Operation.* Final Report, National Highway Traffic Safety Administration, 400 7th St. S.W., Washington, D.C., 20590.

WILDE, G. J. S., J. L'HOSTE, D. SHEPPARD, and G. WIND. 1971. *Road Safety Campaigns: Design and Evaluation.* Paris: Organization for Economic Cooperation and Development.

Chapter 7

ALCOHOL TAXES AND HIGHWAY SAFETY

by Charles E. Phelps

Introduction and Overview

Taxation of alcohol to reduce drinking-related vehicle crashes represents an idea with growing support. Most obviously, higher alcohol taxes generate potentially large federal revenue to offset the large budget deficit. Alcohol taxation not only can produce large revenues, but has the added advantage that it eliminates much economically harmful behavior as well, whereas most other taxes create harmful distortions in the economy. Even after accounting for reductions in consumption that a higher tax would produce, Hacker (1987) estimates that restoring real taxes to their 1950 level and equalizing tax rates across all types of alcoholic beverages would generate $20 billion per year in new tax revenues.

On a more analytic level, the most prominent feature is that the tax rates per alcohol-equivalent dose differ greatly across types of beverage. Distilled spirits ("liquor") are taxed at a higher rate (about $.20 per ethanol-ounce) than beer (about $.05 per ethanol-ounce) or wine (about $.01 per ethanol-ounce). At least two of these beverages are taxed at the wrong rate. This raises the second question: what is the "right" rate of alcoholic beverage taxation? The inflation-adjusted tax has fallen by a factor of four since 1950.

I gratefully acknowledge valuable comments on previous drafts from John Graham and Michael Grossman.

Which era had a tax that was closer to the "right" rate? A discussion of this issue follows.

Thoughts on the "Right" Tax

If the primary policy goal is to reduce alcohol-related crashes, injuries, and fatalities, we must recognize that alcoholic beverage taxation represents a very blunt instrument. We use this instrument poorly now—almost certainly insufficiently—but it surely can and should be employed to reduce alcohol-related vehicle crashes. To understand why taxation is such a blunt instrument requires an understanding both of the relationships between drinking and driving behaviors and those of drinking behaviors and prices.

A key feature of the problem is the hugely nonlinear relationship between alcoholic consumption and propensity to cause vehicle crashes. The apparent increase in risk of a fatal auto accident rises precipitously with blood alcohol level. For young drivers, the risk of a fatal crash is 100 times higher with a blood alcohol level (BAC) exceeding the driving-under-the-influence (DUI) level of .1 percent (Phelps, 1987; Mayhew and Simpson, 1983). For older drivers, a BAC of .15 percent will produce this same increase in relative risk (Mayhew and Simpson, 1983).[1] However, since the absolute risk of fatal accident is so much higher in young drivers than older drivers, the most important group here will remain the youngest drinking drivers. Further, the risks differ greatly depending by daytime and nighttime, quite likely by road conditions, and possibly by the amount of food a person has consumed while drinking.

In all age groups, the risk of fatal vehicle crashes accelerates with BAC. This generates a part of the complexity in devising an optimal tax: mild drinking generates a relatively small increase in risk, even if followed by driving; a considerable amount of drinking that does not precede driving hence creates no added vehicle risk; intensive drinking, coupled with driving, creates massive increases in risk. Any tax rate applied uniformly across all alcoholic beverages must account for this diversity.

Complicating this issue even more is the fact that the relationship between alcohol intake and resultant BAC varies greatly by person. The most obvious relationship comes from body mass— big people *can* drink more than small people and still achieve lower BACs. In addition, while our intuition suggests that some experienced drinkers can "hold their liquor" better than others, no systematic evidence is available to document any such effects.

Combining these phenomena, the incremental expected damage created by a given drink of alcohol depends *at least* on (1) the location of drinking, (2) the total number of drinks consumed, (3) the rate of consumption, (4) the person's body mass and other physical characteristics, and (5) the time of consumption (day vs. night).[2]

The usual economist's prescription says to set a tax on any damage-causing behavior equal to the incremental *external* damage it might cause. Here, the potential problem is highlighted: the expected (average) external damage from a single drink is far lower than the incremental damage *under certain circumstances*. This fundamentally exposes the bluntness of taxation as an instrument to deter drunk driving vehicle crashes. We cannot levy a tax specifically to the conditions of drinking.

A final consideration in this question asks how far the public concern for damage extends. In its most fundamental form, the question centers on how the lives of drunken drivers themselves should be treated. Virtually every analyst would agree that innocent victims of drunk drivers are an externality—a cost imposed by drunk drivers on others. This clearly motivates the imposition of a tax. But how should the lives of the drivers themselves be considered? In my view, this issue turns on the accuracy of knowledge of the drinking driver about the consequences of drinking and driving as combined behaviors.[3]

A comparable (and possibly more complicated) question considers the position of the passenger of a drunk driver. At one extreme, the passenger could be considered equivalently with the driver, under the belief that the passenger can (and should) know the level of intoxication of the driver. At the other extreme, the passenger can be treated as an innocent victim. For reasons that should become clearer below, I tend to treat the passengers as innocent victims in this discussion, but the issue may be moot: some of the evidence available suggests that, for the most part, drivers' deaths should also be considered as an externality.

The following notation will help with this discussion. Suppose that the cost per crash (value lost) is V, and that K represents the average number of "other" persons killed for each alcohol-involved driver killed.[4] If drinkers fully understand the risks of drinking alcohol at various levels, presumably this risk (and the consequences for their own safety) has been incorporated into their demand curves. The observed willingness to pay for alcohol has already subtracted out that risk. Many economists would argue, on the basis that the consumer knows his or her own preferences better than any other person, that self-inflicted damage does not create a role for government intervention. Yet, even die-hard noninterventionists might reconsider this issue in some cases. Consider the question of fatalities alone. In this case, the external damage arising from drinking q drinks is:

$$\text{External damage} = K * V * p \text{ (Dead}|q \text{ drinks).} \qquad (7.1)$$

Alternatively, if the person has no awareness of those risks, then there is an additional "externality" imposed, arising from the lack of information about the risks.[5] Define an awareness level of the *relative risk of drinking and driving* (compared with sober driving) as A, with $A = 1$ being full knowledge and $A = 0$ being the belief that relative risks are invariant with drinking intensity.[6] For any awareness level A, the additional damage (beyond the deaths of "others") unaccounted for by the individual is[7]

$$(1 - A) * V * p \text{ (Dead}|q \text{ drinks)} \qquad (7.2)$$

Then, in general, the external damage is

$$(K + 1 - A) * V * p \text{ (Dead}|q \text{ drinks)} \qquad (7.3)$$

and the *marginal* external damage of the kth drink is

$$(K + 1 - A) * V * dp \text{ (Dead)}/dq \qquad (7.4)$$

evaluated at $q = q_k$.

We can readily see from equation (7.4) that the marginal damage of a drink varies greatly, depending on both the level of awareness (A) and the incremental probability of death following from the kth drink. Particularly since the incremental probability of death accelerates very rapidly with drinking intensity, we must realize that the incremental damage caused by any specific drink similarly varies greatly. This creates a particular problem for the economist who wishes to create a tax equal to the marginal damage—the economist's usual prescription to reduce an external cost.

If a single tax is to be applied across all drinks sold, then it must relate to the average external damage across the possible number of drinks consumed on any given day by a single drinker. This tax must average across both youths and adults, across intensive and light drinking, and across drinking followed (or not) by driving, by day and by night, and across persons with different awareness levels A. These considerations emphasize the complexity of finding the "right" tax for alcoholic beverages.

Any tax levied on any behavior produces a cost, typically measured as the extra value foregone by consumers beyond the price they pay for any commodity or service. If taxes reduce consumption considerably, then the foregone "extra value"[8] can mount rapidly. How fast the loss value increases depends on how price-sensitive consumers' behavior is.

In general, finding the "best" tax for alcoholic beverages involves balancing two "goods": The value of deaths postponed (and injury and property damage) versus the foregone consumer surplus, the "cost" that drinkers pay for foregone value in addition to the taxes they pay for alcohol. The emphasis here on drunk driving deaths by no means implies that these are the only sources of concern from drinking. Alcohol has been implicated in 100,000 to 200,000 annual deaths from all causes (Hacker, 1987). Thus, any steps, including higher taxes, to curtail drinking in general have other benefits as well. But in those other areas of human behavior, much more of the burden falls on the drinkers themselves than on others, raising questions about the role (if any) for government intervention. In vehicular crashes, the externality is so clear and prominent that such questions fall by the wayside.[9]

Previous Studies Relating Alcohol Taxes to Vehicle Crashes

Four studies have attempted to assess directly the effects of alcohol taxes on vehicle crash fatalities. Three of these rely on state-level data, and a fourth combines several different data sets. In this section, I summarize these approaches and results. The next section in the chapter discusses the advantages and disadvantages of each approach for answering the questions at hand.

Studies Using Aggregate State Data

Aggregate state-level studies rely on levels (or changes) in auto fatalities by state, relating them to levels (or changes) in alcohol prices or taxes, often using statistical techniques such as regression analysis to control for other factors that might alter the fatality level.

Philip Cook (1981) provided the first study using state-level data to address the effects of taxes on fatalities. In an ingenious quasi-experimental approach relying on changes in behavior in states where the tax had changed, Cook estimated the effect of higher taxes on fatalities. The median of changes in other states (with no change in taxes) formed the "control group." He estimates that a 10 percent increase in the *price* of liquor would reduce fatalities by 7 percent.[10]

Two more recent studies by Saffer and Grossman (1987a,b) use 1975–1981 data from the 48 contiguous states, and estimate the relationship between beer taxes and highway fatalities.[11] These studies concentrate on the fatality experience of young drivers, and provide age-specific estimates of the effects of beer taxes on fatalities. They estimate the following elasticities of vehicle fatalities with respect to beer taxes:

Age Group	Fatality Elasticity with Respect to Beer Taxes
15–17	−.18
18–20	−.27
21–24	−.19

These results are quite consistent with those of Cook (which aggregate all ages), since one reports the elasticity with respect to price (Cook) and the other with respect to taxes (Saffer and Grossman).[12] The two types of estimates are closely related. Let E_{Mp} = the mortality-rate elasticity with respect to price, and E_{Mt} the elasticity with respect to taxes. Finally, let $s = t/P$—that is, the share of total price accounted for by taxes. Then it will generally be true that

$$E_{Mt} = s * E_{Mp} \qquad (7.5)$$

On average, taxes account for about half of the cost of distilled spirits ($s = .5$) and about one-fifth of the price of beer and wine ($s = .2$). About two-thirds of the liquor tax comes from the federal excise tax, with the remaining third representing the average state and local taxes. State and local taxes account for a much larger fraction of the beer and wine taxes.

Specifically, Saffer and Grossman's estimates of beer price elasticities are consistent with price elasticities in the neighborhood of −1, if the state taxes account for about a fifth of the price of beer.

Studies Using Microdata

One study addresses this problem quite differently, by combining microdata studies of alcohol use with aggregate data on alcohol-related vehicle crashes. In that study (Phelps, 1988), I combined data from a demand study for alcoholic beverages (Grossman, Coate, and Arluck, 1987) with aggregate data on alcohol involvement of drivers who died in vehicle crashes (NHTSA, 1982), relating these data using Bayes' theorem to derive the desired results. Since this approach differs so considerably from the aggregate state-level methods used in all other studies of this phenomenon, a more detailed presentation of this approach follows.

The fundamental questions in controlling drinking-related vehicle crashes are, How does drinking behavior alter the likelihood of a fatal crash? and How does price alter the drinking behavior? The first of these can be derived from existing data, using Bayes' theorem. The second requires specific demand studies.

To learn the relationship between drinking intensity and fatality rates, consider the following relationship. Let p (Death|Drinking level k) be the probability of a fatal crash, given that the person has blood alcohol concentration level k. This is the conditional risk of a fatal crash—the risk we wish to learn. Similarly, let p(BAC level k|Death) represent the likelihood of a dead driver being observed with BAC level k. Such data come, for example, from autopsy studies of drivers in fatal crashes. Third, let the overall probability of a person dying in a fatal crash on any given day be p(Death), readily derived from aggregate fatality statistics reported in the Fatal Accident Reporting System (FARS). Finally, let p(Drinking level k) represent the probability on any given day that a randomly selected person will achieve drinking level k. One source of such data is household survey data, for example.

Given these definitions, it follows from Bayes' theorem that

$$p(\text{Dead}|\text{BAC level } k) = \frac{p(\text{BAC level } k|\text{Dead}) * p(\text{Dead})}{p(\text{BAC level } k)} \quad (7.6)$$

If we can learn each of the components of the right-hand side of equation (7.6), we can then derive the conditional probabilities of death, given any drinking level.

The most difficult of these data to obtain are the unconditional probabilities of a person achieving BAC level k on any day. In Phelps (1988), I adopted the results from a household survey conducted by the National Center for Health Statistics (NCHS), and reported in Grossman, Coate and Arluck (1987). This survey asked individuals (1) how often they drink, and (2) when they drink, how much do they commonly drink? The data were reported in categories of response—for example, for drinking frequency, "daily, 2–3 times per week, . . . , never" and comparably for intensity, "never, 1–2 drinks, 3–5 drinks, 6+ drinks." These data allow an estimate of the average number of persons in the survey who will have a specified number of drinks on any given day, and hence a projection of what fraction of the population will consume that number of drinks on any given day.[13] The final step converts drinking intensity to BAC levels. While (as noted) the relationship between alcohol intake and BAC level varies greatly by person, I used the following conversion in that analysis: 1–2 drinks → 0 <

BAC level < .05; 3–5 drinks → .05 < BAC level < .1; 6+ drinks → BAC level > .1. These levels correspond to the usual legal definitions of alcohol-involved, driving under the influence (DUI), and driving while intoxicated (DWI).

The basic data appear in Tables 7–1 to 7–3, reproduced from Phelps (1988). Using the relationships in Equation (7.6), we obtain the estimates of *daily* risk of fatal vehicle crashes for young drivers shown in Table 7–1.

The estimates of risk levels assume that the propensity to drive remains unaltered, no matter what the level of drinking. If, for example, heavy drinkers drive only half of the distance as sober drivers, then the risk levels are understated by a factor of two (and conversely).

The final step in the analysis links the probabilities of a person drinking (on a given day) and the intensity of drinking with the prices of alcoholic beverages. This requires a still more difficult data problem—the linking of price data to the individual survey data. Grossman, Coate, and Arluck (1987) achieved this using a one-time special survey of alcoholic beverage prices conducted by the Bureau of Labor Statistics (BLS) as a part of its ongoing development of the consumer price index, but appropriate price data are not generally available at present. Their study generated a series of equations estimating the probabilities of these various drinking events (frequency and intensity) as a function of alcohol prices and other variables. In effect, these equations allow estimation of how prices affect the probabilities of drinking—dp(BAC level k)/$d$price. These in turn allow estimation of the effects of higher prices (taxes) on fatalities.[14]

For the age groups 16–21, this microdata approach leads to an estimated reduction in alcohol-related fatalities shown in Table 7–2. This table demonstrates an important phenomenon: the incremental return to fatality reduction falls off as the tax rate rises. Put differently, as some drinking is deterred by higher prices, some

Table 7–1 Alcohol Involvement in Vehicle Crashes for Youths Aged 16–21

	$BAC > .1$	$.1 > BAC > .05$	$.05 > BAC > .01$	$BAC = 0$
Daily Deaths[a]	8.64	1.84	0.95	7.17
Daily Odds[b]	4.55×10^{-5}	4.42×10^{-6}	1.07×10^{-6}	4.62×10^{-7}
Relative Odds (vs. Nondrinker)	98.0	9.6	2.3	1.0

Source: Phelps (1988).
[a]Apportions the 18.64 average daily deaths by blood alcohol levels from Table 7–2, last column.
[b]Ratio of deaths in BAC category to number of youth drinkers in BAC category.

fatalities remain among sober drivers. Eventually, a "prohibitive" tax would still leave a number of fatalities even if it could be enforced.[15] The difference between current fatality levels and this "sober only" fatality rate was calculated by Reed (1981). However (as the next section discusses), this would probably be too high a tax.

The other phenomenon to note is that, at tax rates near current levels, the response of fatalities estimated in Phelps (in press) closely approximates that found by Saffer and Grossman, (1987a) despite the large difference in methods. As noted, they found an elasticity of fatalities with respect to price of about − 1. At a tax rate of 10 percent above current prices, the data in Table 7–2 show a decline in fatalities of about 12 percent, so the elasticity of fatalities with respect to price is about − 1.2. At higher tax rates, the elasticity implied in Table 7–2 falls, eventually to near zero at higher tax rates. As Grossman, Coate, and Arluck (1987) have noted, it should not prove surprising if youths respond more than adults to prices, in part due to the effects of habit formation on adult consumption choices. Thus, the elasticities of fatalities with respect to price, while larger than those found by Cook (1981) (for all persons, for liquor prices) are not unreasonably large.

The Optimal Level of Taxes (and Fatalities)

With estimates in hand of the incremental effects of higher alcohol prices on vehicle-crash fatalities, we can turn to the broader question of finding the "right" tax rate. Following methods similar to those set forth here, I estimated the optimal tax using the results presented above. Then there is a philosophical question that centers on the appropriateness of using "consumer surplus"

Table 7–2   Effects of Higher Beer Tax on Auto Fatalities of Youth Drivers Plus Their Victims

Additional Tax Rate (%)	Total Daily	Alcohol-Related
0	33*	20
10	29	16
20	26	13.5
30	24	12
40	22	8
50	21	4
100	18.5	2

Source: Phelps (1988).
*This corresponds to 18.6 youth driver deaths daily × 1.77 to account for deaths of others.

as a measure of value. Here, I take a classic economist's stance: the consumer is the best judge of how much he values things. Thus, I use the standard measures of consumer surplus in the alcoholic beverage markets to calculate the "costs" of higher taxes on alcohol.[16] The "cost" of such a tax is the foregone consumer surplus (extra value achieved beyond the price paid) on consumption deterred by the higher tax.

As the tax on alcoholic beverages increases, the foregone consumer surplus *increases* at an increasing rate. Since the reductions in fatalities also *decrease* at an increasing rate, there eventually comes a point where a slight increase in the tax rate reduces welfare of the population (consumer surplus) more than is gained (in the value of lost lives). The key questions to implement such a calculation are (1) the value assigned to a lost life[17] and (2) the price responsiveness of the overall alcoholic beverage market, which in turn determines the consumer surplus losses at any tax level.[18] Phelps (1988) calculates the optimal tax under a variety of conditions (different value of life of $1 to $3 million, and demand elasticities for the aggregate market for beer of $-.25$ to -1). Importantly, this study attributes costs for all drinkers, but assumes no gains in fatality reductions arising from higher prices to older drivers. (This occurred because the price responsiveness equations used, estimated by Grossman, Coate, and Arluck (1987), existed only for young drivers.) The optimal tax ranged from 15 to 60 percent of current price, with "most likely" values around 25 to 40 percent. These latter values imply a low level of awareness by youths of the incremental risk, a topic discussed in the next section.

In an extension of this work, Weimer and Vining (1988) made a series of "cautious" assumptions about the effects of a higher alcohol tax on older adult drivers, and also extended the tax to beverages other than beer. They made all of their calculations at a 30 percent tax rate (rather than searching for the optimal tax). A comparison of their results with the fatality effects for young drivers only suggests that the results in Phelps (1988) understate the incremental gains by at least 30 percent. Thus, the optimal tax is surely larger than shown in my previous work.

The Perception of Risk

The microdata analysis reveals an important phenomenon that remains masked in state-level aggregate data analysis: the calculation of relative risks of driving and drinking at various levels. Whether or not consumers perceive this risk accurately becomes (in my view) a central part of calculating the external damage from alcohol-related vehicle crashes. As noted above, if consumers have poor perception of the risks, then presumably they exhibit "too much" willingness to pay for alcohol, compared with an informed consumer, and their deaths in vehicle crashes can be thought of as just as much of an externality as those of innocent victims.

A growing body of work in the psychology literature details how consumers' judgments and decisions under uncertainty differ from the usual economist's model. For example, Hogarth (1975) details how people act poorly as "intuitive statisticians," because their ability to process information is limited. Heuristic judgment mechanisms become common, and anticipations about data that might be received heavily color the actual perceptions of new data. People typically badly overstate the certainty with which they judge probabilistic information—not only are their judgments often biased, but their 95 to 99 percent confidence limits often (over 50 percent of the time) do not incorporate the "true" values being estimated.

In a study of people's perceptions of the risk of dying from various events, Slovic, Fischoff, and Lichtenstein (1982) showed that people overstated the dangers of such "dramatic" risks as tornados, floods, and botulism, while understating the risks of more routine illnesses such as diabetes, cancers, strokes, etc. They showed considerable overconfidence about events over which they believe they have control—for example, driving automobiles.

This literature points toward an important issue in the drunk driving problem: the informed consumer must not only understand the risks of driving a motor vehicle, but also be able to assess how rapidly those risks change as the level of drinking changes. The literature suggests that this sort of statistical estimate will be made quite poorly, and probably with too much confidence.

To investigate this matter, I have conducted some preliminary studies suggesting that, at least for some young adults, the perception of increases in risk from drinking are *far* lower than the actual increases. As I report in Phelps (1987), a survey of undergraduates[19] shows that (on average) they perceive the risk of 6+ drinks at about 7.5 times the risk of sober driving, compared with the actual relative risk of nearly 100. To the extent that these students even approximately represent their cohort around the country, this strongly suggests that the risks of drinking have not been fully incorporated into the decisions to consume alcohol. In the notation used above, the awareness level A is probably much closer to 0 than 1 for these students.

Methodological Dilemmas

Each of the studies discussed above—and many "potential" studies not yet carried out—confront serious methodological problems in their attempts to understand the relationship between drinking and fatal crashes. I briefly review here the strengths and weaknesses of each of these approaches, with the eventual purpose of helping guide future data collection efforts and research strategies.

Aggregate Data

The strengths of aggregate data to study this problem are well known. The highly detailed data on fatal crashes (FARS) provide an excellent measure of the dependent variable for these studies, nationally and state by state, for a long period of time. If the proposed mechanism for altering drinking behavior is the tax, state aggregate data also provide a clear measure of taxes levied in each state, year by year. Since the tax level differs by state, and since states change their tax rates from time to time, the cross-sectional and intertemporal variation provides ample opportunity to estimate the relationship between tax levels and fatalities. Cook (1981) and Saffer and Grossman (1987a,b) have taken advantage of these types of data for precisely these obvious attractions.[20]

Aggregate data are not without defects, however. Particularly when using individual states as the unit of observation, a series of potential defects occur:

- Border crossing (making a "booze run" to a neighboring state) blurs the distinction between consumption (by residents) and sales (by vendors).
- State data invariably rely upon tax data to measure quantities. The profitability of tax evasion (underreporting of sales) makes such measures suspect.
- The severity of drinking laws may be correlated with other factors that also influence drinking (e.g., religious preferences of residents). This can bias estimates of the effects of the laws themselves.
- Analysts must make some assumption about how a change in the tax actually emerges as a change in price. Standard economic analysis suggest that, in a competitive industry, a tax levied at the wholesale level will cause, at most, an increase in retail price on a one-for-one basis. In a monopoly, there can be a higher passthrough rate. Cook (1981) presumed a 20 percent markup on taxes levied at the wholesale level, and

Simon (1966) applied an even larger markup. All of these choices alter the apparent relationship between taxes and drinking as well as the relationship between taxes and fatalities.

Previous studies have addressed each of these issues. The results invariably indicate that these issues are more than minor; they can seriously alter our understanding of the relationship between drinking and fatalities.

Several attempts to control for border crossing have met with only limited success. Wales (1968) found that including "border state" prices almost obliterated any statistical relationship between alcohol demand and price. Smith (1976) used the cheapest border state price as a control variable in his studies of alcohol demand and supply. However, as Cook has noted, all border state prices are relevant: a state may import on one border and export on another, depending on the geography of city location and the prices of neighboring states.[21] In some states, the question of border crossing probably matters only a little, but in others, it can create serious problems.[22]

The problem of tax evasion has been studied only by Smith (1976). He developed a careful model of legal and illegal (untaxed) supply, where the prices in both markets depended in part on the enforcement effort of each state. His work clearly shows the potential importance of tax evasion on the estimated relationships between tax levels and consumption. To the extent that this problem carries over to the question of the effects of taxes on fatalities (which seems plausible), aggregate state data face this additional problem.

Finally, recent work by Saffer and Grossman (1987b) shows that even the severity of drinking laws cannot be naively considered as independent of drinking levels themselves. High fatality rates create more demand for more severe laws, for example. Further, high levels of drinking create opportunities for state tax revenue. Thus, alcohol-related laws and highway fatalities cannot be considered as independent. Estimates that fail to account for this may misstate the effects of extending these more severe drinking laws to other states. Saffer and Grossman demonstrate this phenomenon for minimum-age drinking laws, but no studies have carried out the same type of analysis for state tax levels themselves.

Finally, the previous discussion of macro- and microdata studies shows that some types of information are simply masked in macrodata, most obviously the intricate relationships between drinking intensity and fatalities, and the changes in risk as drinking intensity changes. While these questions may not matter considerably in the understanding of the effects of price on fatalities, the absence of insight from the macrodata studies can hide other opportunities and tools to control the problem that may emerge from microdata studies.

Microdata

The contrasting strengths and weaknesses of micro and macrodata are remarkable for the apparent "role reversals" between the two: the strengths of macrodata are the weaknesses in microdata, and conversely. In microdata, quantity measures are often uncertain, and price data nearly impossible to pull off the shelf. In particular, micro-quantity data often rely on recall and survey, the problems of which can be considerable in this topic. While self-reported drinking behavior is the most common method for gathering such information, it appears to underestimate consumption—for example, when extrapolated to and compared with aggregate production, sales, and international trade data.[23] In comparisons I have made of the NCHS survey data used by Grossman, Coate, and Arluck (see Phelps, 1988), there seems to be some underreporting of beer consumption, compared with estimates published by beer marketing organizations. However, these data are not fully comparable (the NCHS data reported by Grossman, Coate, and Arluck refer to 16- to 21-year-olds, while the industry data refer to 18- to 24-year-olds as a single group), and it is possible that the data are consistent. I have not been able to determine the methods used by the marketing industry to infer drinking participation rates, but whatever methods they use seem to show higher participation by young adults than the original NCHS survey showed. In a more recent NCHS survey, youths reported engaging in some beer drinking at rates over 80 percent higher than the earlier study, in part due to lower real prices during the period of the later survey (Coate and Grossman, 1988). All of these contrasts point to the importance of correct survey methodology.

Price data for microstudies are notoriously difficult to obtain. Typically, the researcher obtains a separate survey of retail establishments to measure prices, and then matches those prices geographically to the respondents of a survey (which gathers consumption and other data). In the study by Grossman, Coate, and Arluck, for example, a special one-time BLS intensive study of prices was used that corresponded closely in time to the NCHS household survey they used.

Such an approach hides a number of problems. First, it does not measure the actual transactions prices of the respondents. Prices of alcoholic beverages vary considerably, even within a single city, and often intertemporally. Thus, "the price" in a city is really a distribution of prices, varying by location, month, and most notably, by quality of beverage.[24] The intensity of shopping behavior by the individual can alter the price received. And border crossing by individuals can create the same problems with microdata that state-level data confront. Finally, this approach typically does not account for on-premises drinking prices, although for some persons, a primary location of drinking is a bar or pub.

Some of the uses of currently available microdata require assumptions than cannot be verified. For example, in my earlier work using microdata, I assumed (for lack of other information) that the propensity to drive remained unchanged, no matter what the level of drinking of the person. In simple terms, if drinkers drive less than sober persons, the actual risks of drinking and driving (together) are worse than I have calculated, and conversely. Similarly, I had to assume, for lack of better data, that the intensity and frequency of drinking were uncorrelated. This can produce some subtle biases in some of the estimates I made, but sensitivity tests suggest that the general results remain reasonably stable over a wide range of assumed correlations of quantity and frequency of drinking. I also assumed that the ratio of total fatalities to driver fatalities was the same for young drivers killed in alcohol-related accidents as for all accidents, all ages of drivers. There appear to be some tendencies for drunk drivers to die more in single-car accidents, suggesting that this might overstate "external" deaths. Conversely, the number of occupants of young persons' cars may exceed the national average. These and other assumptions all cloud at least some uses of microdata currently available.

Finally, and obviously, microdata are more expensive to procure and use than aggregate data. The costs of obtaining reliable microdata vastly exceed the costs of finding and processing available state-level data.

Next Steps (or, "If I Were a Rich Man . . .")

In my view, current research has gleaned much, if not all, of the available information from macrodata relating alcohol taxes (price) to alcohol-related vehicle crashes. The next steps to take in this question will require substantial new microdata gathering, if we really wish to learn more about these relationships. I see data gathering as having several separate (and possibly separable) components.

Consumption and Driving Patterns

To make serious knowledge gains, we will need extensive and reliable data on drinking patterns, showing how much people drink of various beverages, by day and perhaps even by time of day, for all age groups, and for a sufficiently large sample to allow national representation. This same data-gathering effort should gather as much detail as possible on the driving patterns of the respondents, and the associations of drinking and driving. The two basic approaches to gathering alcohol-consumption data are a simple quantity-frequency (QF) approach[25] and a diary (either retrospective or prospective). The retrospective diary commonly covers the previous week (Redman et al., 1987) but has been extended as far as the previous 30 days (Sobell et al., 1982). In one direct comparison of instruments on the same population, the retrospective diary produced a considerably higher measure of total consumption than the QF approach (Redman et al., 1987). The diary method has the other direct advantage of measuring the *pattern* of consumption, providing a much better measure of intense drinking—the most dangerous from the point of vehicle crashes.

To my knowledge, no study has combined a measure of drinking and driving patterns, except at the very crudest level.[26] If the administration proved feasible, I would conjecture that the knowledge gained from a diary-based survey that combined drinking and driving patterns would produce enormous gains in our understanding of drunk driving. Further, I do not see any particular reason why it would be infeasible to administer.

I wish to emphasize the importance of gathering better information on the patterns of drinking and driving, because it may be the only way we can learn enough about these joint behaviors to sharpen the otherwise-blunt instruments we have to control alcohol-related vehicle crashes.[27]

The same sort of survey could potentially gather price information, both by asking what had been paid at retail establishments, and methods to learn prices paid for package beverages. The latter could include either a household inventory, or questions about the retailer from whom beverages had been purchased, or both.[28] The latter approach obviously requires a follow-up visit to the retailer, but it can be undertaken entirely noninvasively and indeed, without any need for cooperation by the retailer.[29]

We should also remember that a survey need not directly measure vehicular crashes of the respondents; drinking and driving behavior patterns will suffice. We can combine such data with auto fatality data through Bayes' theorem to understand the key issues associated with alcohol use and vehicle crashes.

Consumer Perceptions

A separate issue emerges from the earlier work on alcohol-related fatal crashes—the perceptions of consumers about the risks of drinking and driving, and indeed, their knowledge of how drinking activity translates into BAC levels. In my preliminary study of college students, the perceptions of the increase in risk dramatically understated the actual rates, as computed from my study and independently derived with other methods (Mayhew and Simpson, 1983; Reed, 1981). Even with the current intensity of anti-drunk driving campaigns, consumers may still not fully appreciate the risks of the behavior. This suggests an entirely different approach to modifying drinking/driving behavior than "price"—that is, the provision of information.[30] Separate studies, of course, would need to be undertaken to learn the most effective methods for conveying information about risks of drinking and driving.

Most desirably, the same sample would be used to measure drinking and driving behaviors and beliefs about the risks of those conjoint activities. While the "beliefs" information could be derived separately from the "consumption" information, such a separation would eliminate the opportunity to link the behaviors with the beliefs. If the behaviors relate to beliefs, and if changing the beliefs alters the behavior, then the comprehensive survey approach (using the same sample) would be fruitful.

If research supports the hypothesis that behavior is related to beliefs about the risks of drinking and driving, a separate issue then emerges: can changing those beliefs alter behavior, and if so, what is the most effective way to present information to persons to improve their knowledge of risks? These questions have been explored quite extensively in the field of cigarette smoking, with some possible spillovers to the drunk driving problem.

As a brief aside, the legal status of manufacturers' warning bears some mention here. Many states adopt the *Restatement (2nd) of Torts* (American Law Institute, 1965) as the fundamental basis for their legal decisions on liability. In that compendium, manufacturers' liability and duty to warn about product hazards are quite limited: Section 402A, comments h–j, provide the following:

(h) A product is not in a defective condition when it is safe for normal handling and consumption. If the injury results from . . . abnormal consumption, as where a child eats too much candy and is made ill, the seller is not liable.

(i) The article sold must be dangerous to an extent beyond that which would be contemplated by the ordinary consumer who purchases it, with the ordinary knowledge common to the community as to its characteristics. Good whiskey is not unreasonably dangerous merely because it will make some people drunk, and is especially dangerous to alcoholics.

(j) [I]n order to prevent the product from being unreasonably dangerous, the seller may be required to give directions or warning on the container as to its use, but a seller is not required to warn with respect to products, *or ingredients in them, which are only dangerous, or potentially so, when consumed in excessive quantity, or over a long period of time,* when the danger, or potentiality of danger, is generally known and recognized. . . . *again, the dangers of alcoholic beverages are an example. . . . [emphasis added]*

Particularly the last comment (j) emphasizes the role of consumer knowledge. If (as my preliminary studies of young drivers show) persons greatly underperceive the risks of drunk driving, then manufacturers may have a duty to warn under this formulation of tort liability. In general, I would argue that we do not know what "is generally known and recognized" in this area.

Summary

In conclusion, I summarize briefly the points made previously. First and most prominently, the tax on alcoholic beverages should certainly increase; the appropriate level can be further assessed with better studies, but for substantial increases in taxes, the value of reduced fatalities, injuries, and property damage surely outweighs the costs to society. All available evidence suggests that, despite the bluntness of a tax in surgically removing alcohol-involved driving, a higher tax is nevertheless a good idea.

The "right" tax is difficult to estimate with precision at present, because we lack good data on the drinking patterns and responsiveness of adults, and we lack clear understanding of the associations between drinking and driving for all age groups. Better information will greatly reduce such uncertainty, and allow a more careful and precise estimate of how high the tax should be set.

Consumers' own perceptions of risk enter the calculation of the proper tax level, but also introduce significant alternative policy options to taxation. If consumers systematically underperceive the risk, then investments in education, including, for example, effective ways to use warning labels on alcoholic beverage containers, may prove fruitful.

Probably, most of the potential gains in knowledge in this area using aggregate data have already appeared. We will need to turn next to careful microdata analyses to enhance substantially our knowledge about the relationships between drinking, driving, and alcohol taxes. Sufficient research on the validity and reliability of alternative data-gathering methods has been conducted to allow such studies to proceed fruitfully as soon as sufficient funding can be obtained.

Endnotes

1. Reed (1981) reviews a series of studies providing evidence on this subject as well. The evidence from Mayhew and Simpson (1983) is the most complete.
2. This substantial nonlinearity also makes it very hazardous to infer anything about vehicle crashes by assessing the effects of alcohol taxes on aggregate drinking behavior. Two alternative approaches are discussed later in the chapter.
3. I wish to be very specific here: I do not base this discussion on tastes of drinkers, including their preferences for consuming alcohol versus the risks of death, nor any religious or other convictions that might determine their tastes. My discussion focuses on the information they hold, and hence their behavior.
4. NHTSA data show that K is about .77, including passengers of alcohol-related drivers.
5. Michael Wolkoff first suggested to me the importance of incorporating the individual's awareness of risk in these calculations.
6. If a person overperceives the actual risk, then $A > 1$ and such a person would engage in too-little drunk driving. However, evidence I present later suggests quite strongly that this case almost never occurs.
7. The "awareness level" may depend on more than pure knowledge of the probabilities. Recent work in behavioral decision theory suggests that people process information about small risks quite poorly. This can contribute to the reduction of awareness just as the mechanisms I describe in the text. I discuss these issues further below.
8. The economists' term is "consumer surplus," the extra value consumers get beyond the price paid.
9. Alcohol also contributes to more than half of such violent crimes as child and spouse abuse, rape, and homicide (Hacker, 1987).
10. In the usual economists' notation, the price elasticity is $-.7$. Note that to increase the price by 10 percent, the tax must increase by a much greater

percentage amount, since the tax constitutes only a small fraction of the price.

Cook's study used the following methods: for the period between 1960 and 1975, he investigated the changes in automobile fatalities following any change ($.25 per gallon of liquor or greater) in the liquor tax levied in any state. He scales the change in consumption of liquor to the median change in all other states where the tax had not changed (to control for other events that might alter drinking levels). From this, he not only can estimate the price elasticity of demand (his estimate is -1.6) but also the consequent changes in auto fatalities. He calculates the "experimental" change in fatalities in each state in the same way he adjusts the liquor consumption, i.e., by scaling the change in fatalities in each "experimental" state to the median change in comparable-year "control" states.

The most serious potential problem with this study is the belief that changes in the tax rate do not depend on fatalities. If state legislators or regulators believe that their state's death rates have become excessive, they may raise the alcohol tax in response. Thus, the tax rate and the fatality rate would be jointly determined, and Cook's "quasi-experimental" methods could be challenged.

11. Note three differences from Cook's study: he analyzed deaths across all ages. Second, he assessed the effects of a change in prices (not taxes). Third, he studied changes in price of distilled spirits (not beer).

    The approach used by Saffer and Grossman relies on state-level aggregate data, and uses the multiple regression to estimate the effects of alcohol taxes on fatalities, holding other things constant. The "other things held constant" in their studies include (among other things) the legal drinking age in the state, the drinking age of border states, income, vehicle miles traveled, motor vehicle inspection rates, and indicators of the religious preferences of the state's residents.

    One potential problem from their work is the phenomenon of border crossing. States with relatively high prices may find many of their residents purchasing most of their alcohol in neighboring low-price states. Their approach "matches" the auto fatality rates of a state with its own prices. In general, this approach can lead to misestimation of the effect of price on fatalities. However, Saffer and Grossman have attempted to control for this phenomenon, and they conclude that their estimates are not seriously biased by potential border crossing.

12. The elasticity measures the percent change of one variable in response to a 1 percent change in the other. Hence, E_{yx} measures $\%dy/\%dx$.

13. This calculation requires the assumption that drinking intensity and frequency are not correlated. See Phelps, 1988, fn. 18, for a discussion of potential bias resulting from this.

14. The statistical techniques they used are similar to multiple regression analysis, but take account of the discrete nature of the drinking response data being analyzed. The analytic technique—polychotomous logistic regression—allows the researcher to hold constant other variables and assess the separate effect of price on behavior. In the work by Grossman, Coate and Arluck (1987), the other factors held constant included only the price of the various

forms of liquor (distilled spirits, beer, and wine), the legal age of drinking, and the legal drinking age of any neighboring state within 20 miles.

One of the greatest difficulties with their study is the considerable imprecision of some of their estimates. While the estimated effects are often large, they are estimated quite imprecisely, so that the range of possible "true" effects remains large.

15. See R. T. Smith (1976) for a discussion of enforcement issues.

16. A further issue arises here; does the analysis differ depending on whether the drinking consumer is considered in the sober or postdrinking state? Alcohol clearly alters the ability to process information. Thus, a relevant question here asks whether we should assess the behavior of a sober drinker or a drinking drinker?

17. As I show in Phelps (1988), the costs of injuries and property-damage crashes form only a small fraction of the total costs of alcohol-related vehicle crashes when one values lives at levels near or above $1 million.

18. The welfare loss for an incremental tax dt is found by $dW = .5*($spending level$)*(\%dprice)^2*E$, where E is the demand elasticity.

19. The survey was taken among students in my Health Policy class at the University of Rochester.

20. However, in part due to the high quality of work already accomplished here, it may well be that few, if any, further gains in knowledge await us from the use of macro data.

21. A *Wall Street Journal* story some years ago on Cheyenne, Wyoming, provides an example. The story began, "Harry Hoffman's Liquor is a real Cheyenne institution. Everybody in Cheyenne buys their liquor at Harry Hoffman's. The trouble is, Harry Hoffman's is in Denver."

22. Michael Grossman, in work in progress with Gary Becker and Kevin Murphy, provides a measure of the fraction of any state living within 20 miles of each border, and has offered to share this measure with other researchers.

23. Millwood and McCay (1978) conduct such an analysis for the Australian population.

24. For example, "beer" can cost about $.50 per can for low-quality beer (about the same as a soft drink), and upwards of $1.50 per bottle for elite imported beer.

25. This approach asks questions like "When you drink, how much do you typically consume?" and "How often do you drink?"

26. For example, Farrow (1985) has asked respondents if they ever drive after drinking, and the national Health Interview Survey asks "During the past year, how many times did you drive when you had perhaps too much to drink?"

27. As indicated above, the enormous difference between the average danger of a given drink and the conditional danger (in certain situations) leads one to wish for better-aimed instruments. A 30 percent tax on alcohol would have considerable effectiveness. A $100 tax on the 6th drink of a driving person would have far more efficacy. But we do not know how to levy such a tax.

28. In subsequent modeling, the price obtained by individuals will probably vary with drinking intensity, since heavy drinkers have an incentive to search for a low price.

218   *Preventing Automobile Injury*

29. The person conducting the survey would go to the store and sample the prices from the shelf. Since the survey respondents would likely purchase beverages quite near their home, a household visit could readily be followed by a separate trip to the liquor store.
30. In the usual territorial aggrandizement of economists, I will proclaim this as economic turf in addition to "price."

References

American Law Institute. 1965. *Restatement (2nd) Torts*. Philadelphia.

COATE, DOUGLAS, and MICHAL GROSSMAN. 1988. "Effects of Alcoholic Beverage Prices and Legal Drinking Ages on Youth Alcohol Use." *Journal of Law and Economics* 31 (April).

COOK, PHILIP J. 1981. "The Effect of Liquor Taxes on Drinking, Cirrhosis, and Auto Accidents" In Mark H. Moore and Dean R. Gerstein, (eds.), *Alcohol and Public Policy: Beyond the Shadow of Prohibition*. Washington, D.C.: National Academy Press.

FARROW, JAMES A. 1985. "Drinking and Driving Behaviors of 16- to 19-Year-Olds." *Journal of Studies on Alcohol* 46, no. 5.

GROSSMAN, MICHAEL, DOUGLAS COATE, and GREGORY M. ARLUCK. 1987. "Price Sensitivity of Alcoholic Beverages in the United States: Youth Alcohol Consumption." In *Control Issues in Alcohol Abuse Prevention: Strategies for States and Communities, Advances in Substance Abuse, Supplement 1*, pp. 169–98.

HACKER, GEORGE. 1987. "Taxing Booze for Health and Wealth." *Journal of Policy Analysis and Management* 6, no. 4:701–08.

HOGARTH, ROBIN M. 1975. "Cognitive Processes and the Assessment of Subjective Probability Distributions." *Journal of the American Statistical Association*. 70, no. 350 (June):271–89.

MAYHEW, D. R., and H. M. SIMPSON. 1983. "Alcohol, Age, and Risk of Road Accident Involvement." In *Alcohol, Drugs and Traffic Safety*, National Highway Traffic Safety Administration, pp. 937–47.

MILLWOOD, J. E., and A. M. McKAY. 1978. "Measurement of Alcohol Consumption in the Australian Population." *Community Health Studies* 2:123–32.

National Highway Traffic Safety Administration (NHTSA). 1982. *Alcohol Involvement in Traffic Accidents: Recent Estimates from the National Center for Statistics and Analysis*, NHTSA Technical Report, DOT-HS-806-269, May.

PHELPS, CHARLES E. 1987. "Risk and Perceived Risk of Drunk Driving Among Young Drivers." *Journal of Policy Analysis and Management* 6 (4):708–14.

———. 1988. "Death and Taxes: An Opportunity for Substitution." *Journal of Health Economics*, no. 1:1–24.

REDMAN, SELINA et al. 1987. "Agreement between Two Measures of Alcohol Consumption." *Journal of Studies on Alcohol* 48, no. 2.

REED, DAVID S. 1981. "Reducing the Costs of Drinking and Driving." In Mark H. Moore and Dean R. Gerstein (eds.), *Alcohol and Public Policy: Beyond the Shadow of Prohibition*. National Academy Press.

SAFFER, HENRY, and MICHAEL GROSSMAN. 1987a. "Beer Taxes, the Legal Drinking Age, and Youth Motor Vehicle Fatalities." *Journal of Legal Studies* 16 (June):351–74.

———. 1987b. "Drinking Age Laws and Highway Mortality Rates: Cause and Effect." *Economic Inquiry* 25, no.3:403–18.

SIMON, J. L., 1966. "The Price Elasticity of Liquor in the U.S. and a Simple Method of Determination," *Econometrica* 43, no.1:193–205.

SLOVIC, PAUL, BARUCH FISCHOFF, and SARAH LICHTENSTEIN. 1982. "Facts versus Fears: Understanding Perceived Risk." In Daniel Kahneman, Paul Slovic and Amos Tversky (eds.), *Judgement Under Uncertainty: Heuristics and Biases*. London: Cambridge University Press.

SMITH, RODNEY T. 1976. "The Legal and Illegal Market for Taxed Goods: Pure Theory and an Application to State Government Taxation of Distilled Spirits." *Journal of Law and Economics* 19, no. 2:393–429.

SOBELL, L. C. et al. 1982. "Do Quantity-Frequency Data Underestimate Drinking-Related Health Risks?" *American Journal of Public Health* 72:823–28.

WALES, TERRENCE. 1968. "Distilled Spirits and Interstate Consumption Effects." *American Economic Review* 58:853–63.

WEIMER, DAVID L., and AIDEN VINING. 1988. *Policy Analysis: Concepts and Practice*, in press.

220-22

p 197 i

v.s. 2
~~9312~~ ?
3240
3230

qv 13

COMMENTS BY MICHAEL GROSSMAN

Charles Phelps is to be congratulated for his very fine cost-benefit analysis of alcohol taxes and highway safety. His approach is novel in that he computes the optimal tax on beer under a variety of alternative assumptions. Thus he extends previous research in this area which has focused on the actual or potential benefits of higher alcoholic beverage prices and taxes in terms of reductions in alcohol use and motor vehicle accident mortality. I have no negative comments on Phelps's work. Therefore, I would like to underscore the potential effectiveness of increased taxation of alcoholic beverages by comparing the impact of a nationwide minimum drinking age of 21 on youth alcohol use and motor vehicle mortality with the impact of various alternative policies that raise federal excise tax rates on alcoholic beverages. I would also like to add one item to Phelps's agenda for future research.

The comparison of tax and drinking age policies is based on my recently completed research project with Douglas Coate, Henry Saffer, and Gregory Arluck, which was funded by the National Institute on Alcohol Abuse and Alcoholism (Grossman, Coate, and Arluck, 1987; Saffer and Grossman, 1987a, b; Coate and Grossman, 1988). In this research, we present the first set of estimates of the responsiveness of youth alcohol use and motor vehicle death rates to variations in the price of alcohol. In addition, we examine the sensitivity of these two outcome measures to increases in the legal drinking age.

Our research on youth alcohol use employs two data sets: the first and second National Health and Nutrition Examination Surveys (NHANES I and NHANES II), conducted by the National Center for Health Statistics between May 1971 and June 1974, and between February 1976 and February 1980. The results from NHANES I serve as the basis for some of Phelps's estimates. The research on youth motor vehicle accident mortality is based on a time series of state cross-sections for the period from 1975 through 1981. We concentrate on beer prices and beer excise tax rates in the research, because beer is the most popular alcoholic beverage among youths. State beer excise taxes on a case of 24 twelve-ounce cans during the period at issue ranged from a low of 4.5 cents in Wyoming to a high of $2.28 in Georgia.

According to our results with NHANES II (the most recent sample), a federal policy that simultaneously taxes the alcohol in beer and liquor at the same rates and offsets the erosion in the real beer tax since 1951 would have reduced the number of youths who drank beer frequently (four to seven times a week, approximately 11 percent of all youths) by 32 percent during the period of NHANES II and would have reduced the number of fairly frequent beer drinkers (one to three times a week, approximately 28 percent of all youths) by 24 percent. The enactment of a uniform minimum drinking age of 21 in all states would have reduced the number of frequent drinkers by 28 percent and the number of fairly frequent drinkers by 11 percent.

With regard to motor vehicle accident mortality, the drinking age policy would have reduced the number of 18- through 20-year-olds killed in motor vehicle crashes by 8 percent in the period 1975–1981. A policy that fixed the federal excise tax on beer in real terms since 1951 would have reduced the number of lives lost in fatal crashes by 15 percent, while a policy that taxed the alcohol in beer at the same rate as the alcohol in liquor would have lowered the number of lives lost by 21 percent. A combination of the two tax policies would have caused a 54 percent decline in the number of youths killed.

The preceding figures suggest that, if reductions in youth alcohol consumption and motor vehicle accident deaths are desired, both a uniform drinking age of 21 and an increase in the federal excise tax rate on beer are effective policies to accomplish this goal. They also suggest that the tax policy may be more potent than the drinking age policy. Indeed, according to our computations, the lives of 1,022 youths aged 18 through 20 would have been saved in a typical year in the 1975–1981 period if the federal excise tax on beer had been indexed to the rate of inflation since 1951. On the other hand, the lives of 555 youths per year aged 18 through 20 would have been saved if the drinking age had been 21 in all states of the United States.

My most important addition to Phelps's agenda for future research pertains to the addictive nature of excessive alcohol use and possibly driving shortly after drinking. Recent theoretical work by Becker and Murphy (forthcoming) suggests that addictive behaviors can be understood in the context of a rational economic model of decisionmaking over the life cycle. Becker and Murphy show that the demand for addictive goods such as cigarettes and alcohol should be inversely related not only to the current price of the good but also to its past and future prices. Past prices are relevant because they affect past consumption of the addictive good, and an increase in past consumption due to a reduction in past price raises current consumption. The future price is relevant because a reduction in it raises future consumption, which lowers the "shadow price" of current consumption.

Becker, Murphy, and I (1987) have applied this model to the demand for cigarettes using a time series of state cross-sections for the period from 1956 through 1985. A structural demand function is obtained in which current consumption depends on current price and on past and future consumption, both of which are treated as endogenous variables. The Becker-Murphy model predicts that the long-run response to a permanent price change should exceed the short-run response in the case of an addictive good. The empirical results support this proposition. Moreover, our long-run price elasticity of demand for cigarettes of $-.77$ is at the high end of existing estimates.*

Currently, Becker, Murphy, and I are using the same model and data base to fit demand functions for distilled spirits and for excessive alcohol consumption measured by cirrhosis mortality. Similar models can be fit with microdata that contain alcohol consumption at several points in the life cycle. If our results for cigarettes also hold for alcohol, the price elasticity of demand for alcoholic beverages may be larger than estimates contained in existing research.

References

BECKER, G. S., and K. M. MURPHY. Forthcoming. "A Theory of Rational Addiction." *Journal of Political Economy*.

BECKER, G. S., M. GROSSMAN, and K. M. MURPHY. 1987. "An Empirical Analysis of Cigarette Addiction." Working paper, University of Chicago, September.

COATE, D., and M. GROSSMAN. 1988. "Effects of Alcoholic Beverage Prices and Legal Drinking Ages on Youth Alcohol Use." *Journal of Law and Economics* 26, no. 1 (April).

GROSSMAN, M., D. COATE, and G. M. ARLUCK. 1987. "Price Sensitivity of Alcoholic Beverages in the United States." In H. D. Holder (ed.), *Control Issues in Alcohol Abuse Prevention: Strategies for Communities*. Greenwich, Conn. JAI Press.

SAFFER, H., and M. GROSSMAN. 1987a. "Beer Taxes, Legal Drinking, and Youth Motor Vehicle Fatalities." *Journal of Legal Studies* 16, no. 2 (June).

————. 1987b. "Drinking Age Laws and Highway Mortality Rates: Cause and Effect." *Economic Inquiry* 25, no. 3 (July).

---

*Becker, Murphy, and I control for incentives to import and export cigarettes across state lines in response to price or tax differences (the problem discussed by Phelps) using separate measures of incentives to smuggle cigarettes long and short distances. Our short-distance import and export variables take account of all border state prices as well as the fraction of a given state's population that lives near each border state.

COMMENTS BY HAROLD D. HOLDER

I found "Alcohol Taxes and Highway Safety" by Charles E. Phelps to be most useful in a policy discussion of the potential of alcohol taxes to reduce alcohol-involved crashes. Phelps makes important contributions by (1) outlining an insightful econometric model of the relationships of alcohol prices and traffic crashes and (2) describing some of the major methodological issues involving data that are needed to test models of this type and to undertake policy research in this area in general.

I would like to add a few comments and suggestions which I believe are relevant to this discussion of the relative ability of alcohol taxes to contribute to reduced alcohol-involved traffic crashes and thus fatalities and injuries.

Alcohol Prices, Consumption, and Alcohol-Related Problems

As Dr. Phelps notes, alcohol taxes as a policy tool for reducing alcohol-involved traffic problems are quite blunt. Increased retail prices as a result of increased taxes will affect a larger set of drinking behaviors—not just drinking and driving. To me, this requires that we be reminded of a larger purpose for taxes as a means to affect retail alcohol prices.

We know, and Dr. Phelps has carefully reviewed the phenomenon, that alcoholic beverages are price-sensitive. Like any commercial product or service, demand and use of alcohol are related to its relative cost. Alcoholic beverages have had for some years fixed excise taxes (the increase in federal excise taxes for distilled spirits in 1985 was modest) which, when coupled with decreases in production and raw material costs and increases in personal disposable income and competition, have resulted in lowered relative costs. Beer, the preferred beverage of the young, is close to the price of soda in many areas.

Thus the issue for those of us interested in preventing alcohol problems, not only traffic safety problems, is how can alcohol taxes be used to reduce the levels of such problems? When the reduction of alcohol-involved traffic problems is viewed within the context of a larger effort to reduce other types of problems, including birth defects, drownings, burns, falls, assaults, pedestrian injuries and deaths, boating accidents, and family violence, the policy tool is not so blunt. Why is this so?

First, we have known for some time that aggregate levels of alcohol consumption are related to aggregate levels of alcohol-involved problems. As per capita levels of alcohol consumption increase, so do indicators of alcohol problems. Researchers initially noted this relationship between cirrhosis deaths (most often the result of heavy chronic drinking) and aggregate per capita sales of alcohol (Brunn et al., 1975; Schmidt and Popham, 1980). The relationship has been observed in most modern industrialized societies. The finding certainly challenged the popular notion that overall levels of alcohol consumption had nothing to do with heavy dependent drinkers and alcoholics. In fact, since the heaviest drinking 5 percent of drinkers consume 50 percent of the alcohol (Moore and Gerstein, 1981), it is not surprising to find this relationship.

However, given the notion that alcoholics would get alcohol no matter what the cost, alcohol policy did not consider retail price an effective potential prevention tool until Phillip Cook documented the relationship between alcohol prices (using state alcohol taxes as surrogates) and cirrhosis deaths (Cook and Tauchen, 1982; Cook, 1987). This was the first time the price elasticity of alcohol had been linked to a surrogate of heavy, chronic drinking. In summary of this point, it is important to evaluate alcohol taxes as a potential means to reduce heavy, high-risk drinking and the associated consequences not only as a means to reduce alcohol-involved traffic problems but other social problems as well.

Rational Model of Consumer Behavior

One of the characteristics of many econometric models of alcohol consumption, including the one proposed by Dr. Phelps, is that which I would describe as the "rational man" factor. This is included in Chapter 7 under the discussion of drinkers' "perception of risk" of injury or death while driving after (or while) drinking. I wish I could be optimistic about this factor as a potential leverage point for drinking drivers, but I cannot. Why?

First, Dr. Phelps's own reported research demonstrates that young adults (and, for that matter, older adults) make bad estimates of their relative risk of injury or death while driving and have little idea of how alcohol greatly increases the risk. Second, a further confound is that ethanol is a legal mind-altering chemical. Therefore, we have a situation (on the average) where as BAC levels increase, rational decisionmaking decreases. For this rational decision to have its greatest impact, the decision about drinking (given that driving will be involved given an assessment of injury risk) must be made *before* drinking begins. I can assure you that studies of drinking patterns do not support the notion of a priori decisionmaking—the designated driver programs, notwithstanding.

Third, we can better manipulate aggregate drinking and driving events and thus alcohol-involved injuries and fatalities by altering the public's perceived risk of DUI arrest (not risk of injury). This does not support a notion that increased information to the driving public about their relative risk of injury while drinking and driving will have any substantial effect on such behavior. Even if we alter behavior via increased perceived risk of arrest, the effect decays over time due to experience which counters the perception.

The success level of mass media and school-based educational programs to prevent heavy high-risk drinking, including drinking and driving, is quite low (see Moskowitz, in press). I would hesitate to encourage efforts to consider the provision of information to consumers about drinking and driving risks as a means to reduce alcohol-involved traffic problems. Certainly, public awareness of problems tends to lower public acceptance of drinking/driving (the current public attention to drunk driving confirms this). At one time walking drunk was judged to be more serious than driving drunk.

Information about the injury risk of drinking and driving alone, without other prevention efforts, is unlikely to alter such behavior and reduce alcohol problems. People know from experience that crashes are rare events when driving, even when driving after drinking. To know that alcohol increases the risk of crash (a perceived rare event) is unlikely to be compelling.

Drinking and Driving Data

I found Dr. Phelps's discussion of data necessary for the undertaking of more in-depth research in this area to be most helpful. He points out a need for data about drinking and about driving patterns. I agree. However, we do have in hand data which I have found useful in developing dynamic models of alcohol use and alcohol problems, including traffic crashes and fatalities (Holder and Blose, 1983). I refer to the series of roadside surveys which have been done in this country under the old Alcohol Safety Action Projects, other specific research projects such as the Stockton study, the recent roadside project by the Insurance Institute for Highway Safety, the series of Canadian roadside surveys, and those done in other countries. When these surveys provide information about regular drinking behavior and current measured BAC of a stopped motorist, we have a much better understanding of the relationship between personal drinking patterns and likelihood of driving while impaired. For example, the Prevention Research Center is about to undertake a longitudinal study of drinking and driving behavior, personal drinking patterns, and drinking contexts.

I should also point out the existence of some laboratory studies of price manipulation in experimental bars, including the work of Tom Babor at Connecticut, which should be mentioned.

Conclusion

Overall, I believe Dr. Phelps has made an important contribution to our discussion of the potential of alcoholic beverage taxes to reduce alcohol problems in general and traffic injuries and fatalities in particular. While we have good data about the general ability of alcoholic beverage taxes to reduce heavy, high-risk consumption in general, we need much better data about the relative price sensitivity of alcohol for age and gender groups, income groups, and ethnic populations to be better able to establish more targeted and "less blunt" uses of alcohol taxes as prevention policy.

References

BRUNN, K. et al. 1975. *Alcohol Control Policies in Public Health Perspective*. Finland: The Finnish Foundation for Alcohol Studies.

COOK, C. P. 1987. "The Impact of Distilled Spirits Taxes on Consumption, Auto Fatalities, and Cirrhosis Mortality." In H. D. Holder (ed.), *Control Issues in Alcohol Abuse Prevention: Strategies for States and Communities*. Greenwich, Conn.: JAI Press.

COOK, P. J., and G. TAUCHEN. 1982. "The Effect of Liquor Taxes on Heavy Drinking." *Bell Journal of Economics 13* (Autumn):379–90.

HOLDER, HAROLD D., and JAMES O. BLOSE. 1983. "Prevention of Alcohol-Related Traffic Problems: Computer Simulation of Alternative Strategies." *Journal of Safety Research"* 14, no. 3:115–29.

MOORE, M. H., and D. R. GERSTEIN. 1981. *Alcohol and Public Policy: Beyond the Shadow of Prohibition*. Washington, D.C.: National Academy Press, 1981.

MOSKOWITZ, J. M. In press. "The Primary Prevention of Alcohol Problems: A Critical Review of the Research Literature." *Journal of Studies on Alcohol*.

SCHMIDT, W., and R. E. POPHAM. 1980. Discussion of paper by Parker and Harman. In T. C. Hardford, D. A. Parker, and L. Light (eds.), *Normative Approaches to the Prevention of Alcohol Abuse and Alcoholism*. Report of a conference in San Diego, April 16–18. Rockville, Md: The National Institute on Alcohol Abuse and Alcoholism, U.S. Dept. of Health, Education and Welfare, pp. 89–105.

COMMENTS BY LESTER B. LAVE

Taxing vice is universally approved. The virtuous benefit from lower taxes and get to feel they are punishing the depraved. Sinners have the satisfaction of knowing their actions are benefitting society and that these tax revenues keep the virtuous from outlawing their vice. Such situations are an economist's nirvana. Doing well by doing good is especially attractive in an era of large budget deficits and a need for additional tax revenues.

But this line of reasoning appears suspicious, since it seems too easy. If raising taxes on alcohol is such a good thing to do, why haven't we already done it? After all, governments have needed additional tax revenue for as long as people have consumed alcohol; surely all these economic advisers couldn't have missed something as attractive as raising a tax that made almost everyone better off.

Sinners want to feel virtuous in contributing to society, but not too virtuous. Above some tax level, they begin to protest, moonshine appears, and the social consensus falls apart. Building a social consensus for a tax hike requires new data or innovative analysis. Charles Phelps presents such analysis and data illuminating the social costs of drunk driving. The analysis is a contribution. But before signing on to support a tax increase, we must remember that taxes are extremely blunt tools; they cannot accomplish missions (such as reducing collisions and injuries involving drunk drivers) with "surgical precision." This means that the support for a tax increase must rest on several grounds, and the various possible negative consequences must be examined.

These criteria are satisfied for an alcohol tax. The social costs of excess drinking include not only injuries and property damage from drunk driving, but also fires caused by drinkers who fall asleep with lit cigarettes, injuries from fighting and falls, other sorts of violence, and crimes such as rape. In addition, there are a range of chronic diseases, including liver disease. While the social costs of drunk driving are high, they seem small compared to the other property damage, trauma, and disease from excess alcohol consumption. Thus Phelps understates the external costs of excess drinking by a good deal when he examines only the costs of vehicle collisions. An optimal tax on alcohol—one that accounts for external costs—is much greater than Phelps estimates.

Phelps presents data to suggest the proper form of the tax. It ought not to be an ad valorum tax, since there is no evidence to suggest that expensive wines cause more damage than cheap ones or that expensive cognac causes more collisions than cheap vodka. His evidence indicates that beer is the greatest culprit. Thus, the tax should be on the alcohol content of the beverage, with perhaps a supplement for beer and cheap wine.

227

Such a tax would be regressive, whereas an ad valorum tax would be progressive. However, much of the problem of highway crashes comes from drunk teenagers and alcoholics, where beer or other cheap alcohol is the source of the alcohol. These teenagers also appear to have the highest price elasticity, and so a tax would do the most to decrease consumption. If the issue is accounting for the externalities of alcohol abuse, there seems to be no alternative to a tax on alcohol, supplemented with a tax on beverages that supply alcohol at the lowest cost per ounce.

One problem with taxing alcohol to decrease consumption is the evidence suggesting that moderate drinking prolongs life expectancy. Society desires to promote consumption of one drink each day, but to discourage greater consumption. Here the bluntness of taxation as a tool is evident. No current tax scheme could simultaneously promote consumption of one drink each day and discourage greater consumption.

Another indication of the bluntness of taxation is that while consumption should decline, collisions might not. Teenagers and other binge drinkers will be able to find the money, on occasion, to purchase too much alcohol (for any tax within reason). A tax increase will cut consumption on average, but this might do nothing to reduce alcohol-related trauma. Indeed, high alcohol prices would lead teenagers to have less experience with alcohol so that they are even less able to make reasonable decisions and perform when drunk.

Taxation and externalities are the core of economists' domain; they are songs we continue to sing, even after the audience has begun to throw rotten tomatoes. A more important issue is risk communication. Teenagers and others need to learn how impaired their driving is when they have drunk too much. No amount of lecture is likely to accomplish this. Instead, for example, a driving simulator could be made available at teen parties. Let people try to drive through a standard course before they drink and after they have attained a blood alcohol level of 0.1 percent. The number of collisions of forecast injuries will do more to get teenagers to understand the risks of drunk driving than hours of lecture. The next step is to teach each to recognize when too much has been drunk.

Changing behavior requires carrots and sticks, understanding the dangers and punishment for wrongdoing. Deterrence alone doesn't appear to be terribly effective, judging from the experience of the Scandinavian countries. They have severe penalties for driving while drunk, but the penalties do not appear to deter drunk driving. For example, Phelps notes that in 1960, half of those in jail in Finland were there because of driving while drunk.

Baruch Fischhoff, Granger Morgan, and I are attempting to understand risk communication. Under a National Science Foundation grant, we are trying to learn how people think about potentially hazardous situations and what types of information or events change behavior. Many people engage in unsafe behavior because they don't understand quite how hazardous it is. While better risk communication is not going to change all this behavior, it is likely to be effective in changing much of it. Other people know the risks but either make bad judgments or let the situation slip out of their control. Finally, some people decide the risky behavior is worthwhile, despite the risks. For the latter two groups, taxation and better law enforcement are probably the actions most likely to reduce trauma.

For these two groups, rationality is not likely to be a good characterization of the decision process; higher taxes may have little efficacy in reducing collisions. Institutions such as Mothers Against Drunk Driving (MADD) and peer support groups might be more effective than price increases. At a nonrational level, these groups must be provided with a socially acceptable reason to limit alcohol consumption and not drive after drinking too much.

Sophisticated risk communication is used infrequently in attempting to prevent alcohol-impaired driving. So far, risk communication has largely been "shouting down the tube" to teenagers and other high-risk groups: what you are doing is stupid and if you do it, you are stupid and a criminal. Two-way communication is rarely attempted to learn the concerns of those at risk. Instead, risk communication is viewed as getting talented Madison Avenue types to sell safety the way they sell soap. These devices cannot possibly be effective unless they address the questions that teenagers want answered. In addition, they are unlikely to be effective unless teenagers get their questions answered in detail, which requires two-way interaction. Thus, risk communication is much more difficult, time-consuming, and person-intensive than has been admitted.

I conclude that higher alcohol taxes are justified. The tax increases ought to be greater than calculated by Phelps, since he failed to account for crime, other trauma, and disease associated with excess drinking. However, he also failed to account for the beneficial effects of having one drink each day. Higher taxes will lower the average amount of drinking, but might do little to change binge drinking and resulting collisions. Thus, programs giving social support for nondrinking or not driving while impaired are important to supplement a high tax. Along with the increase in alcohol taxes, especially the tax on beer, a program in risk communication is needed. This program needs to address the behavior of binge drinkers and demonstrate in a convincing fashion to those who drink the dangers of driving while impaired.

Chapter 8

EVALUATING THE NEW 65 MPH SPEED LIMIT

by Dana B. Kamerud

Introduction

In the spring of 1987 the 100th Congress narrowly passed a bill that partially rescinds the national maximum speed limit of 55 miles per hour (MPH). Specifically, the new law permits states to post speed limits as high as 65 MPH on interstate roads outside urban areas with populations over 50,000. President Reagan supported the higher limit but vetoed the highway spending bill to which it was attached. When his veto was overridden, the higher maximum limit became law. Within a few months 37 states adopted a 65 MPH limit on eligible sections of road, although eight of these restrict certain vehicles to lower speeds.

Evaluation of this measure will be an important concern over the next few years for several reasons. First, there will be political action from both opponents of the new law and from those who favor extending its provisions. Their debate continues because there is no clear consensus on the national maximum speed limit. Polls on the 55 MPH limit seemed to show support for its continuance, but driving behavior did not. The congressional situation was equivocal, as the repeal measure made it to the floor of Congress only after many years of trying, passed by only a slim margin in the House of Representatives, and could be reversed at any time. Finally, the states, going their separate ways, will each be looking for guidance toward the right decision.

The political uncertainty described above suggests that decisions will be made and that a policy-relevant evaluation could have an impact on them. To researchers, however, that is just the frosting on the cake. Our real interest in this evaluation stems from the fact that no one really knows what the effects of higher speeds will be. Regardless of whether a regulatory change seems likely, we simply want to know what the trade-offs are and whether or not this is good public policy.

In this chapter I will propose a research agenda for such an evaluation. It might take several years of experience with the new law to assess its effects with sufficient precision, especially in the area of accident fatalities where there have been substantial unexplained year-to-year fluctuations in the past. Meanwhile, the agenda can serve as a guide to data collection and methodology development. An agenda can be merely a list of things to be considered, and I will indeed try to list all the things that one would want to know in order to do the job.

Before doing so, however, I will make use of the fact that the "old" national maximum speed limit has itself been the subject of serious evaluation. The following analysis of the 55 MPH speed limit demonstrates a way of organizing the facts we may establish about the new higher limit. It also suggests which costs and benefits are likely to dominate the trade-offs created by the new law, and so helps us set priorities among the many things that we would like to measure.

Value Trade-offs and the 55 MPH Limit

Prior to 1974, highway speed limits in the United States were set by state and local authorities. Main rural roads were commonly posted at 60 MPH, with speeds of 70 MPH or more permitted on most interstate freeways, on some other divided highways, and on the rural roads of certain states. Under the best conditions—for example, daytime travel on the rural interstates—drivers averaged up to 65 MPH, with a sizable fraction exceeding 70 MPH.

Individual driving behavior presumably reflects one's perceived trade-off between safety, cost, comfort, and the risk of a ticket on the one hand and one's desire for expeditious travel on the other. In 1973 the view was that the energy situation, especially our dependence on foreign oil sources, had reduced the socially optimal speed below that found on the highway. Thus in early 1974 Congress imposed the 55 MPH speed limit to conserve energy, as motor vehicles generally use less fuel per mile at lower speeds.

When the "energy crisis" passed, proponents of the limit successfully pointed to the improved safety record that apparently came from having slower and more regular traffic streams. The 55 MPH speed limit was then reaffirmed as a safety measure, and stronger measures were instituted to promote compliance by the states.

Estimating the Effects

Many attempts have been made to measure the effects of the 55 MPH limit as it is enforced in practice and to compare its costs and benefits. The most comprehensive of these is the work of a special committee of the Transportation Research Board, a unit of the National Research Council (NRC). Responding to a congressional request for an analysis of the speed limit and its enforcement rules, the committee produced a lengthy report (NRC, 1984). Among other things, that report provides point estimates or ranges of values for the speed limit's safety, travel time, fuel use, and enforcement cost impacts in 1983. Subsequently, I built upon the NRC findings in order to complete the calculations and explicitly compare the rural interstates to the other roads affected by the 55 MPH limit (Kamerud, 1988). Part of that work is reviewed below.

The numbers I obtained for the rural interstates are reproduced in Table 8–1. I sought to express in 1983 dollars everything except

Table 8–1 Effects of the 55 MPH Speed Limit in 1983

Benefits	
Lives Saved	400 to 500 lives
Accident Costs Averted, Excluding Productivity Losses	$36 to $69 million
Productivity not Lost to Nonfatal Disabling Injuries	$6 to $12 million
Fuel Savings	$430 million
Reduced Vehicle Wear	$0 to $70 million
Costs	
Enforcement and Compliance	$42 million
Travel Time for Commercial Truck and Bus Operations	$703 million
Passenger Travel Time in Light Vehicles and Buses	413 million person-hours
Trade-off Summary	
Money	$164 to $273 million lost
Lives	400 to 500 lives saved
"Personal" Time	413 million person-hours lost

Note: Estimates, taken from Kamerud (1988), represent actual 1983 experience versus the pre-1974 situation.

lives saved and personal travel time. The estimate of lives saved
came directly from the NRC report. The value of the accident
outcomes reduced by the 55 MPH limit represents direct medical,
property damage, and legal costs, plus a share of certain public
expenditures; it is about 28 percent of the analogous figure cited
by the NRC for all roads affected by the limit. In addition, I
estimated productivity losses associated with nonfatal disabling
injuries, using a breakdown of injuries by severity and recognizing
that the average rural interstate injury is more severe than the
average injury elsewhere.

Among the nonsafety effects in Table 8–1, the fuel savings came
directly from the NRC report and are valued here at $1.04 per
gallon, the 1983 pretax retail price. The benefit of reduced vehicle
wear at slower speeds is perhaps the item least documented in the
literature, but I included it in order to give lower speed limits the
benefit of the doubt. The cost of enforcing the 55 MPH speed limit
and assuring compliance by the states was estimated in the NRC
report; here 35 percent of the total has been allocated to the rural
interstates.

Another cost of lower speeds is the extra time it takes to drive a
given distance. Using the NRC report and other sources, I estimated the extra vehicle-hours and person-hours of travel time
jointly by road type and vehicle type. As mentioned earlier, travel
time for car and light truck occupants and bus passengers is kept
in units of person-hours at this stage of the analysis. I refer to this
quantity as "personal" travel time, though admittedly some car
and light truck travel is done by people on business. Lower speeds
in commercial trucking, however, clearly represent an economic
loss, as less output (transportation) is produced from given inputs
of capital and labor. Unlike the NRC report, my paper expressed
this impact in dollar terms. Specifically, I estimated the value of
truck time on the rural interstates in 1983 at about $21 per hour,
and used this value to produce the dollar figure for truck and bus
operations that is shown in Table 8–1.

At the bottom of Table 8–1, the benefits and costs that were
expressed in dollars have been aggregated to produce a summary
in three-dimensional units of money, lives, and personal travel
time. Compared to the pre-1974 speed regime, the 55 MPH limit
involves an expenditure of personal travel time to save lives. In
addition, a money cost must be assessed against the lower limit, as
the trucking and enforcement costs exceed the total of various
monetary benefits.[1]

Assessing Three-way Trade-offs

How can we assess such a three-way trade-off of money, lives, and time? For this task, the "value of life" and "value of time" are useful concepts that, while controversial, do make sense if properly understood. The misnamed value of life, expressed in dollars per life saved, is meant to measure the average value we place on a marginal change in risk. Similarly, the value of time, though expressed in dollars per hour, must refer to travel time increments of the duration associated with the policy under study. In my paper I presented reasons for treating the values of life and time as being both finite and strictly positive.

Given a lack of agreement on the "true" values of time and life, I devised the following method for examining trade-offs without adopting fixed values. To illustrate it, suppose we knew that a policy saved L lives at a cost of T hours plus M dollars.[2] If time were valued at X dollars per hour, the cost per life saved would be $C(X) = (T \times X + M)/L$ dollars per life saved. Hence $C(X)$ is also the policy's break-even value of life when time is valued at X dollars per hour, in the sense that cost-benefit analysis will rule in favor of the policy if and only if it uses a value of life greater that $C(X)$.

Now consider the set of all nonnegative pairs (X,Y) where X denotes the value of time and Y denotes the value of life. This quadrant represents all possible opinions about the values of life and time. If T, M, and L are known for a policy, then $C(X)$ is a linear function of X, and the equation $Y = C(X)$ defines the graph of a straight line with positive slope T/L. The portion of this line lying in the quadrant is a ray that I call the "policy representation graph," as it represents the policy's three-way trade-off in two dimensions.

There are at least two ways to use the policy representation graph. First, the equation $Y = C(X)$ can be rewritten as $L \times Y - T \times X - M = 0$, so it is precisely the set of (X,Y) values for which the net benefits of the trade-off (life-saving benefit minus time and money costs) are zero. Hence, the graph divides the quadrant into two regions, and cost-benefit analysis will rule in favor of the policy only if one uses a "value of time and life point" (X,Y) lying in the region above the graph. In this way the graph bounds the region of value opinions favorable to the policy, with the ray itself representing indifference toward the policy.

In the second application, a number of rays representing different policies are drawn on the same set of axes.[3] Visual inspection then shows which policies have similar trade-offs. Moreover, the "higher" rays correspond to the higher cost (less efficient) ways of saving lives. In this way the graph becomes a tool for policy comparison and cost-effectiveness analysis.

Results and Discussion

Getting back to our data, if the trade-off summary at the bottom of Table 8–1 contained only point estimates, the graph for the institution of the 55 MPH limit would be as just described. The presence of interval estimates, however, leads to an interval estimate for the cost of life saving for any given value of time. Hence, in this case, the policy graph will consist of a band rather than a ray, as shown in Figure 8–1. (If the Y-axis is labeled in millions of dollars, the band consists of points satisfying $(413 \times X + 164)/500 < Y < (413 \times X + 273)/400$.) The interpretation is that the speed limit appears justified if your value point (X,Y) is above the band, unjustified if it is below the band, and indifferent or uncertain if it is within the band.

In the literature one can find value of time estimates in the \$4 to \$8 per hour range. (See Kamerud [1988] for references.) Using

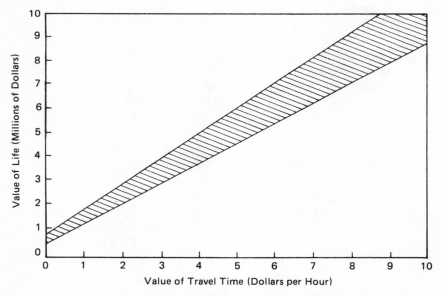

Figure 8-1 Policy Representation Graph for the 55 mph Speed Limit on Rural Interstates, 1983. Axes in 1983 dollars. Shaded band consists of values representing indifference toward the limit as enforced in 1983 versus pre-1974 speeds.

these on the X-axis in Figure 8–1 and projecting to the Y-axis yields a cost of life saving between $3.6 and $8.9 million, which is a good deal more than the cost of life saving attributed to many other highway safety initiatives. Hence, the analysis offers some justification for the repeal of the 55 MPH limit that has taken place.

I also examined the trade-offs for having imposed the 55 MPH limit on the other affected roads (i.e., other than rural interstates) in 1983. For plausible values of time, the cost of life saving there was much less; indeed, it was not out of line with the value of life as estimated in the economics literature. When graphed, the other roads' band (not shown here) fell well below the rural interstates' band. This implies that lives can be saved at far less cost there than on the rural interstates, and so supplies a cost-effectiveness argument for more permissive limits on the rural interstates than elsewhere.

In summary, then, analysis of past experience has been much less favorable toward lower speeds on the rural interstates than on other roads. This means that it could indeed be rational to allow higher limits on the rural interstates, and it would certainly be irrational to do the reverse. The 55 MPH limit seems to have derived relatively more of its costs from personal travel time than from the other net money costs. (According to Table 8–1, each life saved on the rural interstates in 1983 was associated with roughly a 918,000 person-hour time cost plus a $486,000 monetary cost.) Hence, its attractiveness from a societal perspective depends heavily on the values one places on two factors—lives saved by the speed limit and the extra time people must spend in travel.

It remains to be seen what the trade-off picture will be for the new 65 MPH limit. The actual speed increase is likely to be less dramatic than the earlier decrease, when the pre-1974 to 1983 transition cut average speeds from 65 MPH to 59 MPH on the rural interstates. Also, the fatality rate has decreased over the years, so the safety impacts will proceed from a different baseline. Therefore, I do not propose that anyone extrapolate the results for the 55 MPH limit. Rather, the work cited above is a framework that can accommodate information yet to be developed for the new 65 MPH law. The research agenda that follows describes items, methods, and data systems relevant to that task.

Data Needs and Resources for an Assessment of the 65 MPH Limit

The preceding discussion and the publications on which it is based show the types of information that were needed to analyze the

1974–1986 national maximum speed limit. An assessment of the
new legislation calls for a new version of Table 8–1 to describe the
effects of a 65 MPH limit on the rural interstate road system. Past
methods must be adapted to the state-by-state nature of the 1987
legislation, to new estimation techniques, and especially to the
improved data on accidents and speeds available today. These
items are reviewed below, with the critical topic of safety benefit
estimation techniques reserved for the succeeding section.

Safety Effects

To assess the safety effects of a speed limit change, we must
quantify and measure the safety performance of the highway
system before and after the change. The notion of "safety performance" includes the severity, as well as the frequency, of accidents.
Standard data collection practices accommodate this by counting
separately accident outcomes like fatalities, nonfatal injuries (perhaps further categorized by severity level), and property-damage-
only accidents.

A speed change can affect both the frequency and the severity
of crashes. At higher speeds drivers may have some crashes that
previously could have been avoided entirely. Other crashes may
become more severe, perhaps moving to a different category (for
example, from injury to fatal or from property damage to injury).
For this reason the assessment should use a severity scale (where
appropriate) when measuring safety performance with and without
the new speed limit. Data sources for measuring the direct accident outcomes—fatalities, nonfatal injuries, and property damage—are discussed in turn below.

Fatalities. Fatalities play a special role in the trade-off summary
technique I presented earlier and in traffic safety work generally.
In my approach they are dichotomous events, so severity is not an
issue.[4] A complete census of traffic fatalities is available from the
Fatal Accident Reporting System (NHTSA, 1987a) or from the
annual Highway Safety Performance reports and their predecessors
(FHWA, 1987). These data are disaggregated by road type and
state, and the series have been in existence much longer than the
"old" 55 MPH speed limit.

Nonfatal Injuries. The number of injury accidents and the
number of people injured by state and highway type (e.g., rural
interstate) are reported by the Federal Highway Administration
each year (FHWA, 1987). These figures originate with a census of
police reports in each state, with state participation mandated by
federal law (Section 207 of Public Law 97-424). This series, with

its predecessors, goes back to 1967. An alternative source of injury frequency data is *Accident Facts*, where the category most nearly matching the rural interstates is "rural controlled-access" (National Safety Council, 1986). This latter source has a different, more restrictive definition of an injured survivor: it counts only those with disability beyond the day of the accident.

As mentioned earlier, nonfatal injuries should be counted with respect to an injury severity scale like the Abbreviated Injury Scale (AIS). Unfortunately, no national census exists with this level of detail. Instead, for national-level estimates of severity, one must depend on sampling or on extrapolation from certain state data.

One on-going study based on sampling already exists—the National Accident Sampling System, or NASS. NASS collects highly detailed data on a sample of police-reported accidents in each of a number of primary sampling units (PSUs), which are political territories like a city or a group of adjacent counties. The sampling design involves two stages of selection: choosing the PSUs to cover and choosing the sample of accidents within each PSU. Both stages are examples of "unequal probability" sampling.

For example, to generate the 1985 sample, the United States was divided into 1,279 PSUs, which were then grouped into 50 categories described by geographic region, urbanization, and other variables. With selection probabilities proportional to their 1977 populations, one PSU was chosen to represent each category, and teams were sent to these 50 PSUs. The police-reported accidents within each PSU were then sampled using unequal probabilities designed to insure that enough of the more severe (but less frequent) accidents were investigated. In the end the investigators, each averaging about two accidents per week, gathered data on 13,153 of the roughly 6 million police-reported accidents that occurred in 1985 (NHTSA, 1987b).

Injury severity can be measured in several ways from the NASS data. Malliaris, Hitchcock, and Hansen (1985) mention three options. In the first method, each injured survivor is assigned the highest AIS score (1 to 5) of any of his lesions (injuries). In the second, each injured survivor gets a bivariate score describing his two most serious lesions (for example, a person with an AIS-3 head injury and various AIS-1 and AIS-2 injuries would be scored as a (3,2)). In the third method all lesions are counted individually without regard to the number of people carrying them. The first method, called the maximum-AIS or "MAIS" score, is by far the most common. It also offers the advantage that, for each nonfatal MAIS score (1 to 5), the average economic costs per injured traffic accident survivor have already been estimated (NHTSA, 1983).

Is NASS applicable to the problem at hand? In a word, yes. Some of the PSUs are located in states that have already increased their speed limits, so before-after comparisons of the injury severity distribution are theoretically possible, though limited by sample size considerations. Some PSUs are in states that are not presently inclined to change their speed limits, which holds out hope for a comparison of severity changes over time for adopting (65 MPH) states versus nonadopting (55 MPH) states. Not every state contains a NASS primary sampling unit, however, so this remains to be seen. In general, for research on state-by-state policy interventions, it will be helpful if NHTSA keeps the same PSUs from year to year.

Certain states provide an alternative source of nonfatal injury severity data. In some states the police record apparent injury severity when they investigate an accident, often using a three-point scale instead of the AIS. Using the published annual reports of such states, one could estimate the distribution of injuries over the various degrees of severity, conditional on the speed limit. (The design could employ before-after data from states adopting the new limit or, with somewhat stronger assumptions, data from both adopting and nonadopting states.) Then the severity distributions could be used to apportion the FHWA's injury totals over the degrees of severity, separately in adopting and nonadopting states, to get a view of the injury situation allowing for changes in severity as well as frequency.

Dollar Costs of Injury Accidents.   Once the changes in fatalities and in injuries (counted by severity) have been estimated, it remains to convert all the costs except lost life to dollars in order obtain an analogue to Table 8–1. I suggest using a special government report (NHTSA, 1983) for this purpose. For each degree of injury (fatality and MAIS-1 through MAIS-5), that report estimates the average 1980 costs for medical care, legal fees, property damage, and so forth. These components now need to be updated to the study period using appropriate price indices.

Property Damage.   Turning to the matter of property damage, note that losses occurring in fatal and injury accidents have already been estimated in dollar terms, per involved vehicle and by MAIS (NHTSA, 1983). Hence, the remaining problem is to estimate the dollar damages in property-damage-only (PDO) accidents. Once again, there are different data sources for accident frequency and for accident severity (in this case, the average dollar loss per accident).

Police reports are a basic source of PDO accident frequency data. Even if the police are not called to the scene, all crashes with damage over a certain dollar threshold are supposed to be reported. The threshold varies from state to state. Although some accidents go unreported, especially when only one vehicle is involved, this should be less of a problem for research on high-speed roads like the rural interstates.

For the assessment, we desire a tally of PDO accidents by year, state, and road system. Unfortunately, Federal Highway Administration publications do not cover PDO accidents. The state figures may, however, be collected somewhere in the federal government for internal purposes. For example, NASS presumably needs something like this to determine the expansion factors it applies to make national estimates from its unequal probability sample.

One could conceivably obtain this information directly from the state authorities. Fortunately, the National Safety Council (NSC) already gathers the figures, adjusts them for underreporting using unpublished state-specific formulas, and publishes the national total (by road type) each year in *Accident Facts*. The NSC's state subtotals could well be the best source for PDO accident counts by state and road type. Again, there may be a small problem with definitions, as the NSC uses "rural controlled-access" rather than rural interstate.

Finally, PDO accident severity must be measured in dollars and should include items like legal fees and insurance claim administration costs in addition to the damage actually done to vehicles and fixed objects. For all PDO accidents, the cost per damaged vehicle was estimated in 1976 and updated and corrected to 1980 in the study mentioned earlier (NHTSA, 1983). This figure could be further updated using an appropriate price index. Also, I suspect that the average damages per accident are greater on a high-speed road system than overall. I have shown elsewhere how much more costly the average injury is on the rural interstates than overall (Kamerud, 1988). One might just mark up the overall PDO accident cost by the same factor to get a plausible approximation.

Is there a more direct way to estimate the average cost of a PDO accident in a given (possibly future) year and speed regime? NASS deals with property damage in physical rather than economic terms, so it does not offer much help. The insurance industry, through its claims files, is perhaps best able to address this question. In any case, it is worth repeating that higher speeds will not necessarily increase the average loss, because greater crash impacts may push what would have been PDO accidents into the injury categories.

Caveats. Apparently, some sections of what is normally considered the rural interstate system are not eligible for a speed limit increase. From the accident data sources described earlier, one can tell if a fatality or injury occurred on the rural interstate system, but perhaps not whether it was on the portion affected by repeal. The FARS and NASS variable "posted speed limit" might be an acceptable fix. Otherwise, one could proceed as though the change were in effect everywhere on rural interstates in a state that adopted a 65 mph limit. In fact, since there is likely to be behavioral carryover from changed to unchanged sections in the same state, it might be a good idea to do so.

Nonsafety Effects

Analyzing the new 65 MPH limit will also require measurements and parameter estimates for its nonsafety effects, as discussed below. For some of these items, rather little is known and specialized research is in order. For others, better information is available now than was available for the 55 MPH limit studies.

Speeds. Vehicle speeds on the rural interstates need to be measured in both the 55 MPH and 65 MPH situations. Ideally, one would like a vehicle fleet's speed distribution, not just its average speed, in order to calculate its rate of time consumption per vehicle-mile of travel. For small increments to already high freeway speeds, however, this rate is a nearly linear function of speed. Hence, little error would be introduced by using the weighted-mean speeds directly. The travel time benefit achieved by higher speeds is thus approximated by total travel multiplied by the difference between the reciprocals of the mean speeds of the old and new speed distributions. For the accounting format leading to Table 8–1, this approach should be applied separately to speed data for cars, trucks (by size), and buses, if possible.

In addition, before and after speeds are also needed for estimation of the fuel consumption and vehicle wear effects. Moreover, these data can also be used to insure that speeds have not been changing in the nonadopting 55 MPH states, which could be a problem for the regression method of safety change estimation to be discussed later in the chapter.

Where can one find such before and after speed data? As evidence of compliance with the national maximum speed limit, each state is required to monitor speeds on a sample of 55 MPH roads and report the results to the Federal Highway Administration. Since 1982, the measurement sites and procedures have met standards designed to produce more accurate and representative estimates of true driving behavior (NRC, 1984, pp. 28–29). Hence, we have reasonably good estimates of speeds in the "before" period prior to the change to a 65 MPH limit.

The recent federal legislation permitting higher speeds does not, however, mandate similar procedures for the new 65 MPH zones; indeed, the states are no longer required to observe speeds there. For purposes of research, speed reporting must continue on the roads re-posted to 65 MPH. Both NHTSA (a federal agency) and the American Association of State Highway and Transportation Officials (representing the state governments themselves) have called for such voluntary reporting, and the Federal Highway Administration expects that most states will do so. If not, Congress could require it at minimal cost to the federal government, as the federal compliance department for the 55 MPH limit will remain in place. Also, many states have automatic measuring devices embedded in the pavement at key sites, making it inexpensive for them to continue monitoring there.

Enforcement Costs. Expenditures to enforce a law are among the costs associated with its adoption, and should not be reduced by the government's income from fines. (Fines are transfers, not benefits.) We seek the speed limit enforcement cost for rural interstates as a function of speed limit. A higher limit corresponds to reduced enforcement and a benefit here, but this effect will be difficult to estimate. The NRC committee investigated this issue for the 55 MPH limit (NRC, 1984); perhaps the sources it used provide a basis for estimating the continuing cost of enforcement in the nonadopting (55 MPH) states.

In any case, the evaluation should include costs arising in a state's court and fine-collection systems, those in its speed-monitoring and compliance systems (a relatively minor component in the NRC study), and time costs for citizens delayed in their travels or making court appearances, in addition to the more obvious police-related costs. It is not necessary to assume that police patrols are reduced overall. Rather, what is desired is an estimate of the net benefits of redeploying police resources from speed enforcement to other activities.

Fuel Consumption Costs. The effect of higher speeds on motor fuel expenditures cannot be measured directly. Rather, it must be derived from the vehicle speed data in two stages, the first to estimate how much more fuel is used and the second to value that fuel in dollars. In both stages we need updated estimates reflecting the vehicle characteristics and fuel prices of the period under study.

How does speed affect fuel consumption? Although the speed versus fuel economy relation varies from car to car, sources suggest that a 10 MPH increase in highway speed will increase average passenger car fuel consumption by about 15 percent.[5] It is common to operate a 1983 vintage car at 30 miles per gallon or 0.0333 gallons per mile (GPM) at highway speed on level roadway (NRC, 1984, Table A-29; and Holcomb, Floyd, and Cagle, 1987, Table 2.21). Hence, a 10 MPH speed increment increases fuel consumption by (0.15) (0.333) = 0.005 GPM. Assuming linearity, this implies a fuel consumption sensitivity rate of 0.0005 GPM per MPH.

In the past, values as high as 0.0009 GPM per MPH have been used (Jondrow, Bowes, and Levy, 1983), but the difference may simply reflect fuel efficiency improvements over time. (See Table A-29 of NRC [1984] for estimates by model year.) The NRC report itself never explicitly forms the GPM/MPH ratio, but its derived figures for all vehicles on rural interstates imply a sensitivity of 0.0005 GPM per MPH, the same as suggested above for cars alone (NRC [1984], Tables 52 and A-23).[6] In the absence of updated tests, this parameter value may yield our best estimate of extra fuel consumption, provided that the speed change can be measured accurately.

For the second stage, the evaluators must decide the dollar worth of each gallon of motor fuel. Elsewhere I have presented the case for using retail price minus excise tax to value fuel at the societal level (Kamerud, 1988). This choice is not universal: some economists give petroleum a marginal social cost higher than its market price, citing externalities associated with dependence on foreign sources. In any case, it is easy to repeat the assessment using different unit values for motor fuel.

Vehicle Wear.   The NRC report mentions the idea that higher speeds may result in greater vehicle wear and maintenance per mile of travel (NRC, 1984, p. 117). Apparently, there is very little information with which to quantify this claim, so for now this remains an agenda item for the engineering community. For a discussion of the assumptions one might use to produce an estimate from various published figures, see Kamerud (1988).

Truckers' Value of Time.   A higher speed limit should improve productivity in the transportation industry, conferring a monetary benefit on society. Elsewhere I used data from the early 1980s to estimate the value of time for commercial truck and bus operations in 1983 (Kamerud, 1988). My calculations captured driver compensation and opportunity costs, and were adapted to the specific mix of truck types found on the rural interstates versus the other affected roads. By the time the 65 MPH limit can be evaluated, this dollar-per-hour value will need updating, too.

Techniques for Safety Impact Estimation

For most of the topics discussed in the preceding section, it is obvious how to apply the parameter values, impact estimates, or "before" and "after" data pairs to the accounting framework leading to Table 8–1. Safety impacts are, however, an exception to this statement. They depend on how the safety performance observed in states with the new speed limit compares to what would have happened there under the old lower limit. But estimating "what might have been" in a dynamic field like traffic safety is not a simple matter.

For one thing, the analyst must deal with "encountered" data. Political realities will not allow a designed experiment, like applying the new law only to a randomly chosen half of the states next year and only to the others the year after. Our federal system does encourage public policy experiments, but I doubt that any voters who have been craving higher limits will sacrifice this bit of autonomy to the goal of research.

With an intervention of this sort, one might be tempted simply to compare the "before" and "after" periods in the adopting states, or compare adopting and nonadopting states at a point in time. The first of these study designs could be biased by not paying due regard to past trends, while regional differences in population, economy, and travel behavior could threaten the validity of the second. Moreover, even if the adopting and nonadopting states had many similar characteristics, legislative decisions are nonrandom and self-selection bias could result.[7]

The methods surveyed below seek to control for trends and for differences between the states, though they do not completely eliminate the possibility of bias. Each method represents specific assumptions, strengths, and weaknesses—important technical issues discussed in greater detail in the chapter by Garber (1988). Although they address minimum legal drinking age laws, Garber's opinions are relevant to the study of other safety-relevant policies with state-by-state adoption, including speed limits, legal driving age, seat belt and motorcycle helmet use laws and so forth.

Some General Concerns

Before applying an estimation technique, one must decide whether to measure impacts with a *count* of adverse outcomes or a *rate* like deaths per vehicle mile of travel or annual accidents per licensed driver. A simple comparison of counts would miss the role travel activity plays in the accident-generating process. Nevertheless, predictions can be made by using counts as dependent variables in regression models (especially if travel is among the explanatory variables) or in autoregressive trend-extrapolation models.

The use of rates per vehicle mile is an attempt to capture exposure right from the start. Moreover, measuring safety this way embodies the (perhaps not universal) view that our concern with any technology ought not to be "how safe," but rather "how safe per unit of output." One problem with rates is their dependence on travel volume estimates produced by methods that vary across states, road systems, and time. Another issue is that a comparison of rates would implicitly assume that accidents are proportional to travel, or at least that accident changes are proportional to travel changes.

Another general issue for the evaluator is defining the 55 MPH "before" and 65 MPH "after" periods. In most states the new speed limit became effective sometime in mid-1987, so the changes do not correspond with calendar year data. A simple solution is to forget 1987, using 1974–1986 as the "before" period and 1988 and later as the "after" period. Another solution is to include the effective dates in one's modeling. This requires great care, however, because both travel and accident rates vary significantly with the seasons of the year. Since the other explanatory variables might not fully capture these seasonal variations, one would need to add dummy seasonality variables to the model specification.

Multiple Regression Models

This method can apply to any collection of roads adopting the new speed limit, an obvious choice being the set of all rural interstates that make the switch. The idea is to explain mathematically the numbers or rates of adverse outcomes on these roads as functions of various explanatory variables, using data from the 55 MPH period. Then the values of the explanatory variables measured in the "after" period are used as inputs to the model, producing an estimate of what would have happened if the speed change had not occurred.

Data. The first issue is what sample to use for model construction. Most commonly, a time series of annual data is used. In our problem there would be only 13 data points representing the 55 MPH experience from 1974 to 1986. Monthly data exist for accident counts, travel volumes, and most economic indicators, so one could use monthly time series instead, perhaps interpolating those variables that are measured only yearly. In addition to time series samples, the traffic safety field has also seen cross-sectional studies using the 50 states as data points and combined cross-sectional/time series data sets (see Garber [1988] for citations), both possibilities here.

Functional Form. A number of choices exist for the functional form of the regression equation. As mentioned above, one can measure safety performance with either counts or their corresponding rates. With time series data, the measurements can then either be kept as levels or replaced by their first differences. (In the latter case, the explanatory variables would probably need to be differenced, too.) Still staying within the linear model framework, one can then specify either an additive model for the dependent variable or the equally common multiplicative model (additive model for the logarithm of the dependent variable). With today's computer packages it is feasible to try all of these options. One can even use Box-Cox procedures to let the data itself select a transformation of variables.

Explanatory Variables. Next, the explanatory variables must be chosen. If predicting numbers of outcomes instead of rates, one must include exposure (e.g., vehicle miles of travel) as an explanatory variable, possibly in a nonlinear role. Overall economic conditions are another determinant of safety performance. Not only does economic growth increase accidents by stimulating travel demand, but it also seems to increase the fatality rate per mile driven.

One proposed explanation for needing to include economic conditions even after accounting for aggregate travel is that in good times more discretionary travel (partying, cruising, vacationing) occurs, and the young have improved access to cars. Hence, measures of economic activity like real gross national product (GNP) should help explain the accident *count*, while changes in them should help explain the accident *rate*. Alternatively, differencing might be in order to explain the accident rate. For example, a percentage rise in GNP exceeding that in travel might indicate an accident rate increase due to proportionately more discretionary driving. We've gone through a couple of turns of the business cycle since the 55 MPH limit was enacted, which should help us produce good estimates of the impact of the economy on accidents during that period.

A large number of other indicators have appeared as explanatory variables in past models of traffic accident generation. These include levels of employment and unemployment; fuel price and "energy crises"; demographic variables (like the fraction of drivers who are in a certain age group); per capita purchases of beverage alcohol; the average vehicle mass of the fleet; the fractions of travel done by motorcycles and by heavy trucks; traffic density (vehicle miles per road mile); the estimated extent of seat belt use; and that old reliable catch-all, "trend." Any new regression model will be criticized by someone if it fails to let all of these contend.

Nevertheless, some of these forces won't have their full usual effects on the rural interstates. Others will be redundant, having already been captured in the general economic or trend terms. Still others really don't measure what we want them to (like alcohol not measuring drinking-driving). Hence, it is not enough to plug this all in and "let the data speak." The regression analyst should also discuss these issues and review the plausibility of any coefficient estimates advanced.

Model Adequacy.   Goodness of fit to past data must be checked, but that is only necessary, not sufficient, to convince readers about regression-based estimates of what might have been. Here the states not adopting the new speed limit can play a role. Keeping the same functional form and explanatory variables, the regression model's parameters can be reestimated with pre-1987 data from the nonadopting states. Then one can examine that model's ability to predict post-1988 results there. The final test is how the errors of estimation compare, in size and direction, with the effects we claim to be measuring in the adopting states.

Autoregressive Models

Many regression studies use socioeconomic explanatory variables representing contemporaneous "causes" of accidents and have the goals of parameter estimation and theory testing, not prediction itself. Here our interest is predicting what the accident count or rate would be if the speed limit had not changed. Prediction from a time series can be done in another way, with autoregressive models that use the accident results of past time periods as explanatory variables. Rather than trying to identify the causes of accidents, one merely assumes that they change slowly enough to permit prediction from past trends. Finally, one can also add traditional explanatory variables to the autoregressive model, with the criterion for inclusion being added predictive power, which is stricter than the statistical significance criteria of straight regression studies.

Anyone planning such an effort should note the study by Hoxie, Skinner, and Wang (1984), an investigation of socioeconomic factors that one might use to make annual or month-to-month step-ahead forecasts of the total highway fatality count in the United States.

Appropriately for our problem, it used data going back only to 1975. The results were: (1) out of 34 socioeconomic indicators and after much testing and fitting, only a few showed signs of Granger causality, and (2) in prediction tests there was no statistically significant evidence that any of these few "causes" added power to the baseline autoregressive model.

Unlike this pure prediction problem, the speed limit evaluation will be able to use coincident explanatory variables. For example, 1989 economic conditions can play a role in our estimate of what 1989 fatalities would have been without the speed change. Nevertheless, the examination by Hoxie, Skinner, and Wang (1984) suggests that an autoregressive model augmented by a few coincident variables like travel and economic conditions might do the best possible job of prediction. The issue will then be how the expected prediction errors compare to the impacts of the change to 65 MPH. Once again, an appeal to the roads keeping the old speed limit can be made.

Treatment-Control Approaches

In exchange for certain assumptions, treatment-control approaches offer a much simpler way to estimate differences between what occurs with the new speed limit and what would have occurred if the old one had been kept. These methods can be applied to event frequencies (fatality and accident counts) or to other numerical outcome variables like fatality rate and total collision costs.

Although the terminology and underlying problems are similar, what I propose here is *not* the classical premeasure-postmeasure design used in medical and educational research. There the treatment and control groups are sets of individual, equally weighted observational units, usually people. Here the two groups will be collectives of exposure situations, like sections of road or aggregates of travel. I also propose to estimate relative (not absolute) differences, performing a multiplicative (not additive) type of adjustment. Nevertheless, the insights about the problem of confounding in premeasure-postmeasure designs found in Chapter 12 of Anderson et al. (1980) are applicable here.

The Method. As an example, consider Table 8–2, a two-way breakdown of counts with roads defining the treatment and control groups. The idea is to compare the percentage change in the treatment group to that in the control group. The assumption is that (b/a) is the fatality change ratio corresponding to no change in speed limit, due to whatever other factors are present.[8] Hence,

Table 8–2 A Treatment-Control Matrix for Fatality Counts

	Before the Change (pre-1987)	After the Change (post-1987)
Treatment group (change)	limit = 55 Observe a^* fatalities	limit = 65 Observe b^* fatalities
Control group (no change)	limit = 55 Observe a fatalities	limit = 55 Observe b fatalities

without the change we would have expected the treatment group to have $(b/a)\,(a^*)$ fatalities instead of b^* fatalities.

Table 8–2 thus suggests that the speed limit change altered the incidence of fatalities by a factor of size k = observed/expected = $(b^*)/[(b/a)\,(a^*)]$ = $(a)\,(b^*)/(a^*)\,(b)$, which is the reciprocal of the cross-product ratio of the table. If $k = 1$ we see no change; if k exceeds 1 we are claiming an increase; and so forth. As an example, if fatalities in the control group were up by 6 percent and those in the treatment group were up by 14 percent, then the estimate would be that higher speeds increased fatalities by 7.5 percent (because $1.14/1.06 = 1.075$).

Making National Estimates. This is really a common technique that has been used recently to estimate the effects of seat belt laws and of changes in the drinking age, and there are several ways to apply it to the 65 MPH speed limit. Taking all adopting rural interstates together to form the treatment group is the simplest and most natural application. What, then, should be the control group? For a road-specific, state-specific speed limit increment there are several choices, each representing roads with no speed limit change. The rural interstates of all nonadopting states and the other rural arterial roads of the adopting states are two appealing ones for this example.

Table 8–3 suggests five different controls, each of which provides an estimate of treatment effect for the adopting roads. Actually, each control could give two estimates, one by using counts and another by using rates per vehicle mile of travel. One might include the observed percentage changes "c" in the table to summarize the range of behavior; they are not part of the calculations. For ease of comprehension, I suggest reporting percentage estimates of treatment effect "e," where $e = (k - 1) \times 100\%$, instead of the ratios "k" themselves.

For assessing safety impacts at the national level, I have suggested using all affected roads as the treatment group and either the nonadopting rural interstates or the adopting states' rural arterials as control groups. Less attractive control choices include

Table 8–3 Suggested Format for Displaying Multiple Estimates of a Treatment Effect

	Fatalities or Fatality Rate			
	Observed Behavior (Count or Rate)		*Percent Change*[a]	*Indicated Percentage Effect*[b]
	Before	*After*		
Treatment group:				
rural interstates				
in adopting states	a*	b*	c*	0%
Control groups:				
Adopting states				
other rural arterials	a	b	c	e%
urban interstates	–	–	–	–
Nonadopting states				
rural interstates	–	–	–	–
other rural arterials	–	–	–	–
urban interstates	–	–	–	–

Note: Treatment group represents pooled national experience. Example shows how five control groups give five estimates of the percent change in fatalities or in fatality rate.
[a]The observed percentage change is given by $c = ((b/a) - 1) \times 100\%$.
[b]The indicated effect is given by $e = [(a)(b^*)/(a^*)(b) - 1] \times 100\%$ and represents the effect of the speed change on the treatment group for each choice of control group. The column of alternative e-values is the point of the table.

other states' rural arterials and urban interstates in either group of states. Unfortunately for research, if most states adopt the new limit, the nonadopting rural interstates will represent only a small sample of accidents. In general, allowing noninterstate roads to join the control group brings in more exposure and accident experience, though happenings on such roads are less relevant to policy on the rural interstates. Nevertheless, if the preponderance of states adopt 65 MPH, we may have to allow nonrural interstates into the control group.

Single State Estimates. Some state legislatures might also ask for state-specific safety impact assessments. A version of Table 8–3 can be constructed for a single adopting state by using its rural interstates as the treatment group and the following as the control groups defining the rows of the table: other rural arterials or urban interstates from the state in question; various systems (rural interstates, other rural arterials, or urban interstates) for all nonadopting states collectively; and (if possible) the rural interstates of a neighboring nonadopting state. I suggest using its other rural arterials if you are not afraid of speed carryover from one system to another in the same state, and the rural interstates of nonadopting states if you are.

The "paired states" method is also attractive. It requires two otherwise similar states, of which exactly one adopts the new limit. This is essentially the old "Vermont versus New Hampshire" approach so popular among political scientists. Ideally, the states should be neighbors, and not too different: Kansas versus Nebraska would make sense; California versus Nevada would not. It may be hard to find similar neighbors who take different positions regarding the speed limit. (I have seen a photograph of the governors of Minnesota and Wisconsin changing highway signs to "Speed Limit 65" at the same ceremony; no chance for any comparative research there!)

There is yet another reason for making single state estimates. Suppose each adopting state's treatment group was compared to a fixed control group (like the combined rural interstates in all nonadopting states) to produce a set of similarly estimated *"e"* values, one for each adopting state. The dispersion of these derived impact measures would be of interest, and we would be gratified if they were not too diverse. Moreover, a global estimate of *"e"* can be found by weighting and combining the individual estimates. This sort of thing has been done in the past in a very similar context, namely that of changes in motorcycle helmet wearing laws (Chenier and Evans, 1987).

Sources of Bias. What problems can bias the estimates from this treatment-control method? First, something that affects safety (population, traffic volume, economic conditions, or the presence of other safety initiatives) could happen to change more in one group of states or roads than the other. Knowing this would help us decide what to use for the control group. One partial fix is to control for exposure by using rates per vehicle mile in the table instead of counts. (Error in the measurement of travel is always a concern when such rates are used, but fortunately the treatment-control method ultimately depends on only the before-to-after percentage changes in travel, and not on the absolute levels.)

In addition, there is the possibility of self-selection bias, as the adopting states were not chosen at random. A state with a worsening safety record, or even just a poor record of safety improvement vis-à-vis the others, might keep the lower limit because it feels it needs the extra regulation. If trends continue, the 55 MPH group gets an adverse addition. This is the bias direction suggested for drinking age laws by Saffer and Grossman (1987). The opposite would occur if an adopting state's willingness to deregulate epitomizes the same attitudes that cause a relatively bad safety trend. If trends continue, the 65 MPH group gets the adverse addition.

Western states with above-average fatality rates will be among those sure to adopt 65 MPH. This need not be a biasing self-selection as long as the higher rates existed before as well as after the change. Supporters of lower speed limits always point to the confluence of high speeds and troubling safety records in such states, but that doesn't prove anything about the effects of the *change*.

The possibilities raised above (namely, changes in a recognized causative "something" and self-selection) are sufficient, but not necessary, to cause trouble. In premeasure-postmeasure studies one can have bias when, for whatever reason, the outcome variable is changing in the absence of the treatment, especially if it is changing at different rates in different individuals or groups. (See Chapter 12 of Anderson et al. [1980].) Fortunately, in the traffic safety area one can observe whether the treatment and control groups were in similar trends in the past.

A Safety Research Agenda

A credible assessment of the new speed limit's safety impacts may have to wait until we have a year or more of experience with it, but much can be done in the meantime. The work of Hoxie, Skinner, and Wang (1984) and other authors must be adapted to the problem of predicting status quo future accident rates from 1974–1986 data. Although most past studies dealt only with fatality rates, models for nonfatal injuries and property damage are also needed for this project and in general. There has been some discussion of how to estimate what the impacts will be (Hoskin, 1986). Someone should look into the likelihood that they will be detectable.

Once the data arrive, the treatment-control method can produce quick results to compare to those arising from prediction models. It would be desirable for the outputs of these various methods to come out together instead of dribbling into the press. Having seen some rather bizarre press reports already, however, I doubt that this will happen.

Going beyond the new legislation, other areas of speed limit policy need the attention of safety researchers. One of these is fine-tuning our speed limits for safety and mobility. Reformers are already asking for 70 MPH in some rural areas and 65 MPH on more roads than are presently authorized. Similarly, the research community should be looking at variable day/night speed limits and car/truck speed limits. Also at issue are ways to improve safety within the high-speed zones, like warning drivers when they should slow down and teaching lane discipline ("lane courtesy") as in Europe. Research on all of these could be going on in parallel, now.

So far, my suggestions have been oriented to a policy analysis taking the societal view. Accidents have been depicted as the undesired by-products of an otherwise productive sociotechnical system, with speed limits seen as one of the controls on that system. Indeed, most of the sessions of this conference concern systemic controls—laws, regulations, and practices that apply to broadly defined groups of drivers. Our tools have been aggregate data, statistics, and economics; our focus has been on safety policy evaluation and improvement.

An in-depth study of actual rural interstate accidents would be an interesting alternative. As described earlier, the data are available. For fatalities there is FARS, and a population of about 1,800 fatal accidents (2,200 fatalities) on rural interstates each year. For accidents in general, there are NASS and the accident files of certain states. The safety literature provides many ideas of what to look for: impaired drivers, drivers with previous accidents on their records, weather, breakdowns, construction zones, night driving, and so forth.

Often in public health work such a study of "cases" provides a new perspective. Trying the clinical, as well as the epidemiological, approach could reveal how much of the problem has a specific cause and how much is due to systemic background factors. By better identifying the leverage points and better quantifying the impact of countermeasures, one might avoid putting broad-brush solutions on isolated problems.

Summary

The following propositions regarding evaluation of the new law permitting speed limits up to 65 MPH on rural interstate highways have been advanced:

- The author's previous study of the 55 MPH speed limit identifies the various costs and benefits and provides a framework for viewing the resulting trade-off.
- New data sources will permit more accurate measurement of speed limit effects than was possible with the 55 MPH limit.
- If the National Research Council's findings for the 55 MPH limit are applicable, the trade-off will turn on the fatality risk and personal travel time effects, and hence on one's values of life and time.

- For purposes of research, speed monitoring should be continued on the 65 MPH roads as well as on those still posted at 55
  MPH.
- When sufficient data become available, several methods
  should be used for safety impact assessment and the results
  compared.
- Though not strictly necessary for the analysis, an in-depth
  study of rural interstate accidents would be welcome.

Some of the observations made here should also be applicable
to other traffic safety policies that create money-life-time trade-offs
or that are implemented on a road-specific or state-specific basis.

Endnotes

1. This last statement apparently holds for the rural interstates but not for the
   collection of other affected roads—see Kamerud (1988) for details.
2. For the switch to 55 MPH on the rural interstates, it appears that M is positive;
   for other policies M could be negative with no change in the technique.
3. Imagine one for a lower speed limit on rural interstates, another for the same
   on other roads, another for abolishing right turns on a red light, another for
   mandatory vehicle safety inspections, and so on.
4. Severity *is* sometimes discussed in relation to fatalities; e.g., when victim
   demographics are invoked to describe the impact of traffic deaths. Current
   readers so inclined can simply adjust their value of life opinions accordingly.
5. See, for example, Cope (1973), Baerwald (1976, page 27), NRC (1984, Table
   A-27), and Holcomb, Floyd, and Cagle (1987, Table 2.21).
6. The figures were 414 million gallons of fuel annually from a 6 MPH speed
   reduction and 140,778 million vehicle-miles of travel.
7. In the analogous situation of drinking-age laws, research suggests that a poor
   safety record encourages tighter regulation and that ignoring this endogeneity
   produces biased impact estimates (Saffer and Grossman, 1987).
8. This assumption is questionable if higher speeds carry over from adopting
   roads to the control group, one reason why future compliance with 55 MPH
   limits is still interesting.

References

ANDERSON, SHARON, ARIANE AUQUIER, WALTER W. HAUCK, DAVID OAKES,
WALTER VANDAELE, and HERBERT I. WEISBERG. 1980. *Statistical Methods
for Comparative Studies: Techniques for Bias Reduction*. New York: John Wiley
& Sons.
BAERWALD, JOHN E., ed. 1976. *Transportation and Traffic Engineering Hand-*

book, Institute of Transportation Engineers. Englewood Cliffs, N.J.: Prentice-Hall.

CHENIER, THOMAS C., and LEONARD EVANS. 1987. "Motorcycle Fatalities and the Repeal of Mandatory Helmet Wearing Laws." *Accident Analysis and Prevention* 19, no. 2 (April):133–39.

COPE, EDWIN M. 1973. *The Effect of Speed on Automobile Gasoline Consumption Rates*, Final Report, DOT-FHWA-53136. Federal Highway Administration, October.

Federal Highway Administration (FHWA). 1987. *Highway Safety Performance—1985: Fatal and Injury Accident Rates on Public Roads in the United States*. Annual Report to Congress pursuant to Section 207 of Public Law 97-424, HHS-22/7–87 (1M600) QE, Washington, D.C., May.

GARBER, STEVEN. 1988. "On Statistical and Quasi-Experimental Methods to Evaluate the Effects of Minimum Legal Drinking Ages on Highway Safety." Chapter 5 of this volume.

HOLCOMB, MARY C., STEPHANIE D. FLOYD, and STACY L. CAGLE. 1987. *Transportation Energy Data Book: Edition 9*, ORNL-6325, Oak Ridge National Laboratory, Oak Ridge, Tenn., April.

HOSKIN, ALAN F. 1986. "Consequences of Raising the Speed Limit." *Journal of Safety Research* 17, no. 4 (Winter):179–82.

HOXIE, PAUL, DAVID SKINNER, and GEORGE H. WANG. 1984. *Socio-economic Influences on Highway Fatalities: An Empirical Investigation*. Final Report, DOT-TSC-NHTSA-84-1, NHTSA (Washington) and Transportation Systems Center, February.

JONDROW, JAMES, MARIANNE BOWES, and ROBERT LEVY. 1983. "The Optimum Speed Limit." *Economic Inquiry* 21 (July):325–36.

KAMERUD, DANA B. 1988. "Benefits and Costs of the 55 MPH Speed Limit: New Estimates and Their Implications." *Journal of Policy Analysis and Management* 7, no. 2:341–52.

MALLIARIS, A. C., RALPH HITCHCOCK, and MARIE HANSEN. 1985. "Harm Causation and Ranking in Car Crashes." SAE Technical Paper 850090, Society of Automotive Engineers, Warrendale, Penn.

National Highway Traffic Safety Administration. 1983. *The Economic Costs to Society of Motor Vehicle Accidents*. DOT-HS-806-342, Washington, D.C.

———. 1987a. *Fatal Accident Reporting System—1985: A Review of Information on Fatal Traffic Accidents in the U.S. in 1985*, Annual Report, DOT-HS-807-071, Washington, D.C., February.

———. 1987b. *National Accident Sampling System—1985: A Report on Traffic Accidents and Injuries in the United States*. Seventh Annual Report, DOT-HS-807-074, Washington, D.C., February.

National Research Council, Transportation Research Board. 1984. *Fifty-Five: A Decade of Experience*. Transportation Research Board Special Report 204, Washington, D.C.

National Safety Council. 1986. *Accident Facts, 1986 edition*. Annual report, Chicago.

SAFFER, HENRY, and MICHAEL GROSSMAN. 1987. "Drinking Age Laws and Highway Mortality Rates: Cause and Effect." *Economic Inquiry*, 25 (July): 403–417.

COMMENTS BY FRANK A. HAIGHT

I am pleased to be asked to comment on "Evaluating the New 65 MPH Speed Limit" by Dana Kamerud. Three aspects of the work seem to me to be praiseworthy, and I would like to discuss each briefly.

First, the work embodies objective research. The title of this conference emphasizes *both* research and intervention (i.e., "prevention"), but in most traffic safety studies, intervention goals overwhelm research and seriously bias methodology. The justification of some countermeasure program is often an acknowledged or implicit purpose of research and thus any conclusions that may emerge lack an important prerequisite for scientific validity: objectivity.

By restricting our studies to those designed to justify interventions, we deprive ourselves of a reliable knowledge base. It is worth noting that traffic safety is not unique in this respect. According to a currently popular book—*Chaos*, by James Gleick—even hard science can suffer from overemphasis on control at the expense of knowledge. Speaking of investigations of turbulence, the author writes: "Practical interest in turbulence has always been in the foreground, and the practical interest is usually one-sided: make the turbulence go away"; he goes on to explain that this is a contributing factor to our relative ignorance of turbulence. The parallel with traffic safety is striking.

Without wishing to slight the importance of safety interventions, it seems to me that there is also a need for pure research. Just as in biological science, where bacteriology coexists with hygiene, it should be possible, in my view, for disinterested scientific investigation of safety to coexist with countermeasure programs.

Specifically, in Kamarud's work, I am pleased to see an analysis of speed limits, which is designed neither to favor 55 MPH nor 65 MPH, but only to devise a method for measuring the consequences of either. Perhaps the author has an opinion about which speed limit is preferable, but he certainly did not disclose his preference here.

The second reason for praising Kamarud's work is that it explicitly recognizes the trade-off between safety and mobility. Unlike some other hazards to health, such as smoking, transportation has a positive purpose and an economic value. An analysis that ignores this purpose is difficult to take seriously. Any number of countermeasures would clearly "save lives" at the expense of transport performance. As a not entirely trivial example, consider a class of roads which provides a *zero* fatality rate—deep sand roads. Although the safety payoff would be hard to deny, we would scarcely consider building all our roads of deep sand.

257

The choice of a speed limit is a type of intervention in which the effect on mobility is relatively straightforward. Nevertheless, some effect is also implicit in belt-wearing laws, drinking-age legislation, and even in alcohol-related countermeasures. Research which shows only the safety-related consequences of an intervention is, by definition, incomplete. This is easy work to do, since virtually anything that restricts mobility will contribute to some extent to safety. The serious problem is to estimate how much the contribution will be in comparison with the mobility costs, and this is what Kamerud tries to do.

Finally, the work is noteworthy for its methodology. The author takes a first step toward showing *how* to carry out an objective, mobility-sensitive analysis of a particular subject: speed limits. The mobility side of the ledger is expressed both in time and in money, and the trade-offs are built directly into the model.

It is true that Kamerud's basic parameters (value of time and of life) are fairly crude. In the future it will surely be possible to devise more sophisticated measures with which to characterize the mobility-safety balance. Nevertheless, the manner in which Kamerud uses these quantities represents a significant advance in accident research, and points the way for other investigations.

259-62   U.S.

92-13 92-12

9/60

COMMENTS BY JUDITH LEE STONE

Dana Kamerud's objective seems to be to provide a research/ evaluation methodology for the speed limit change. It is difficult to focus on statistical techniques when common sense and the naked eye tell you speeds are creeping up and fatality numbers are rising. As a nation we seem to have a kind of "national schizophrenia" about speed as a risk factor, and new evaluation methodologies won't get it back on the worry list where it belongs.

Kamerud's work begins with the premise that "no one really knows what the effects of higher speeds will be," and as background he describes the pre-1974 patchwork quilt of speed limits and average speeds. That early experience alone gives us a basis for comparison and, coupled with the experience from 1974 to 1987, we have a clear indication that higher speed limits will translate once again into higher speeds and increased fatalities and injuries. I find the premise to be a little faulty.

In the discussion of value trade-offs, the author refers to lost travel time in commercial trucking as a clear representation of economic loss, "as less output (transportation) is produced from given inputs of capital and labor." On the face of it, this might appear true and logical, but the American Trucking Association's fact sheet in support of the lower limit states otherwise:

Since 1974, the American Trucking Association has supported the 55 MPH national speed limit for the following reasons:

- *Data show that the severity of truck-related accidents have decreased since inception of the 55 MPH speed limit.*
- *55 saves fuel. One of our larger member companies estimates that they save $1 million per month in fuel costs by drivers traveling at 55 instead of 60 MPH.*
- *55 extends the life of the vehicle and components.*
- *55 reduces the effects of "splash and spray" in bad weather— one of the major complaints about trucks by passenger car drivers. There is no substitute for simply slowing down to curb this problem.*

I would add other research that documents the fact that drivers are less fatigued at the end of a trip at consistently lower speeds.

The figures from Table 8–1, estimating the effects of the 55 MPH speed limit in 1983, seem very low. By the author's admission, there is a given lack of agreement on the "true" values of time and life, and I maintain it is difficult at best to break out all these values for rural interstates only.

In the discussion of three-way trade-offs, Kamerud concludes that "analysis of past experience has been much less favorable toward lower speeds on the rural interstates than on other roads.

This means that it could indeed be rational to allow higher limits on the rural interstates, *and it would certainly be irrational to do the reverse"* (emphasis added). I hope this was simply a poor choice of words, or researcher's jargon, because I think the statement and conclusion ignore a whole rash of rational and irrational factors that would point to a different conclusion. These are exactly the kind of comments that are quoted out of context by opponents of the speed limit.

I think Kamerud makes an excellent point about the need to continue monitoring both the new 65 roads and the old 55 roads. He cites AASHTO as one group calling for voluntary reporting, although just this week that organization passed a resolution at its annual meeting calling for cessation of monitoring on 55 roads. States in the New England region, many of which have stayed at 55, offered the resolution to create a more equitable situation vis-à-vis federal sanctions. Many of those states feel they are being penalized for taking the safer position, as they must continue to report to the federal government, risking sanctions, and the states opting to go to 65 are not required to monitor or report on the 65 MPH roads. I think it is simply a matter of time before Congress reinstates the requirement that states submit monitoring data from the 65 roads to the federal government.

As regards the research agenda, additional research is needed on speed limits preferred and chosen by older drivers. By the year 2010, 20 years from now, 25 percent of drivers will be over the age of 65.

Current Environment and Challenges Ahead

A few short days ago, at the annual conference of the American Association of State Highway and Transportation Officials (AASHTO), some alarming preliminary data on the recent effect of raising the maximum speed limit in Nebraska and Missouri were presented. In Nebraska, state engineers have seen a 53 percent increase in fatal and injury crashes since the speed limit was raised, with speeds on urban interstates rising, and a 75 percent increase in work-zone accidents. A Missouri transportation official spoke of an 11.2 percent increase in accidents on rural interstate, or 65 MPH roads, while urban roads actually enjoyed a decrease. A representative from the state of Georgia, a state still at 55 MPH but surrounded by states at 65 MPH, warned on the same panel that speed and fatal injury trends both statewide and at state lines are up. All presentors were worried about the direction in which this data seem to be going.

California was represented on this same panel, and claimed that the 65 MPH limit has had no demonstrable effect on safety. Its spokesperson admitted the 55 MPH limit is probably good for safety, but said "limits are flexible things," and should be a reflection of public response. (If we were to follow that line of reasoning in setting all highway safety policy, we would be compelled to raise the legal blood alcohol content limit to .18 because most drunk drivers don't like it at .10, or we should only enforce safety belt laws for adults and babies because teenagers don't like to wear them.)

NHTSA will soon release its preliminary speed data showing a similar alarming upward trend in speeds and fatalities. The Insurance Institute for Highway Safety research has documented New Mexico's experience, showing 61 percent of all cars now going faster than 65 MPH, and nearly 100 percent of cars and trucks exceeding the 55 MPH limit on urban interstates.

If one agrees that speed *at any level* is a major risk factor in motor vehicle crashes—and most responsible people do—then the challenges for the future are to improve both the messages delivered and received throughout the society on this issue, and the quality of leadership in public and private sectors. We often hear that the message out of Washington for the last six years has been that it is a social disgrace to drink and drive, but it's perfectly OK to speed. "Leave your belt off and you're a dummy, but go ahead and speed." We seem to have lost, perhaps released control of, the issue that speed is a major risk factor.

Another major mixed message comes from the "high-tech" and automobile industries (primarily the foreign manufacturers). The front cover of the Sharper Image catalogue glamorizes the ultimate fuzz-buster, and a recent BMW ad touts its product as the best excuse for "tripling the speed limit." The National Association of Governors' Highway Safety Representatives (NAGHSR) passed a resolution at its annual meeting last month urging manufacturers to examine advertising policies on "muscle" and high performance vehicles, as to how they affect the public's perception of the importance of speed.

Many suggest beefed-up enforcement as the solution, but enforcement of the kind we need to see is not possible in the days of budget cuts. We have put so many new traffic safety laws on the books, so quickly, that we do not have the administrative machinery, or the political commitment or will, to make them all effective. We lack sufficient public policy to back up vigorous enforcement

and the public understanding that is essential for obtaining voluntary compliance. If we leave speed off the list of issues the motoring
public should be wary of, we will continue to see upward trends in
fatalities and injuries due to increased speeds, and a deterioration
of the progress gained through vigorous drunk driving and occupant protection law enforcement.

Chapter 9

THEMES AND FUTURE DIRECTIONS

by John D. Graham and Eric Latimer

In this final chapter, the conference chairman and the rapporteur offer their interpretation of the major themes of the conference and attempt to fashion a coherent research agenda from the many and varied contributions that were made. Given the diversity of values, ideas, and perspectives expressed by the participants, we are forced to emphasize some themes, interpretations, and suggestions at the expense of others. We trust that the "benefits" of a conference summary will justify the inevitable arbitrariness that occurs when complex discussions are summarized.

Major Conference Themes

One of the major goals of the conference was to draw scientists, practitioners, and advocates together in a forum where both substantive injury control issues and methodological challenges in evaluation research could be assessed from multiple points of view. Several major themes emerged from the conference discussion. First, injury control countermeasures that aim to alter human behavior deserve more serious attention than they have received in recent decades. Second, the tension between scientific rigor and political advocacy should not be allowed to disrupt progress toward injury control, since both orientations are compatible. Third, while the injury control community is represented by people who hold different values about the proper role of government, some injury prevention strategies can be heartily endorsed by the entire community. Finally, analysts responsible for evaluating injury control policies should do a better job of using alternative statistical methods to examine the robustness of their findings. Each of these four themes is discussed in some detail below.

The Resurgence of Behavioral Interventions

One of the historic debates in traffic safety policy pits those who advocate technological or vehicle-oriented countermeasures against those who advocate driver- or behavior-oriented countermeasures. Obviously, both types of countermeasures can be effective to some extent, but there are divergent opinions about which strategy will prove to be most productive in the long run and where the neglected opportunities are.

In the first half of the 20th century, the traffic safety establishment (police, insurers, physicians, and car makers) concentrated on improving driver performance. This emphasis resulted in driver education and training programs, licensing standards, new traffic laws and law enforcement campaigns. The safety revolution of the 1960s, spearheaded by Daniel Patrick Moynihan, Ralph Nader, and William Haddon, Jr., proceeded from a growing realization that the emphasis on driver-oriented countermeasures had contributed to a neglect of vehicle-oriented countermeasures (e.g., see Moynihan, 1959; Nader, 1972). The 1960s and early 1970s spawned a proliferation of vehicle safety improvements, especially crashworthiness features such as padded dashboards, safety belts, safety door locks, and energy-absorbing steering columns. Many of these crashworthiness features appear to "pass" both the public health and cost-benefit tests (GAO, 1976; Robertson, 1981; Graham, 1984; Crandall et. al, 1986); air bags and automatic belts are expected to produce further benefits.

The chapters in this book indicate a resurgence of interest in behavioral countermeasures in the 1980s. Laws requiring use of child restraints have been adopted throughout the country, and the recent proliferation of adult restraint use laws has been remarkable. Legislative, enforcement, and judicial policies aimed at deterring drunken driving have been widely embraced, while social norms about the acceptability of drunk driving appear to be changing. Policy debates are no longer about whether drunk driving should or can be curtailed but about which countermeasures will be more effective: for example, higher legal minimum drinking ages or increased alcohol taxes. Meanwhile, the trend toward relaxed speed limits is being watched carefully by auto safety advocates and the police for evidence of increased injury counts.

Thus, it is now abundantly clear that both behavioral and technological interventions can be effective. Society's intellectual challenge is to identify the portfolio of technological and behavioral countermeasures that will best achieve reductions in injury yet not exceed society's limited resources for this area.

Science and Advocacy

Conference participants repeatedly raised the issue of the proper roles of science and advocacy in injury control. Although these activities are not always consciously distinguished by participants (it is often difficult to do so!), it became apparent that there was a societal need for both enterprises and that they needed to be separated and nurtured yet ultimately combined in public policy.

A strong sentiment expressed at the conference was that there were too few pure scientists in traffic safety—people who sought to advance theories, test them against data, and develop new methods. In the ideal, the primary goal of such scientists is to acquire and communicate an increased understanding of the processes that produce injuries and the interventions that might prevent them. Like medical researchers, they may view their ultimate goal as helping to save lives and mitigate injuries, but they are sufficiently disengaged from the political process to be reticent about making policy pronouncements. If such pronouncements are made, they are done so on the basis of the scientist's best assessment of the evidence. Even if the scientist would on occasion play an advocacy role, he or she would take pains to be very clear about when the science ends and the advocacy begins.

At the same time, a strong sentiment was expressed that advocacy of injury control is not necessarily in conflict with scientific pursuits. The advocate draws on science in deciding what problems to place on the agenda, what policies to advocate, and what evidence to advance in support of various positions. Advocates also help define the scientific agenda by influencing how much research is funded, which research topics are funded, and which research questions scientists tend to find interesting.

While science and advocacy are compatible, they are surely not identical. The advocate's role is to make the strongest possible case for a position in the context of a pluralist process. Injury control desperately needs advocacy in a society deeply concerned about cancer, AIDS, and environmental pollution—let alone economic productivity, deficit reduction, and Star Wars. In this context, a dispassionate dissertation on the strengths and limitations of injury control is likely to be far less effectively politically then an arousing press briefing on the tragedy of injury and neglected prevention opportunities. Injury control advocates, like all advocates, do not necessarily view it as their responsibility to expose the weakness in their political arguments. They rely on their opponents in the adversarial political process to help lay out all the evidence and the full range of positions.

In short, science and advocacy are different yet compatible and mutually supportive. Injury control advocates need scientists to help them decide what to advocate and what arguments and evidence to advance in support of their positions. Likewise, scientists need injury control advocates to help shake loose societal resources for their work and to help shape research agendas that are responsive to societal needs. While the norms and intellectual orientations of advocates and scientists may seem to be incompatible, both activities have a critical role to play in the growth and maturation of injury control.

Alternative Value Frameworks

As argued in Chapter 1, any piece of research that purports to evaluate an injury control policy must embrace (implicitly or explicitly) one or more value frameworks. Throughout the conference discussion, it was apparent that there was no consensus about which value framework should govern evaluation of traffic safety countermeasures. The disagreement is not surprising in light of the profound ideological and philosophical cleavages in our society at large.

For the most part, conference participants seemed to rally around either a public health framework or a cost-benefit framework. The public health ethic asks policy evaluators to analyze interventions exclusively or primarily in terms of their effects on injuries. Although some public health advocates are supportive of attempts to measure the economic costs of injuries to society, their preferences among policy alternatives tend to be driven toward those that do the most to lessen the incidence and severity of injuries—without regard to cost. In contrast, the cost-benefit ethic asserts that injury reduction is only one of many "goods" valued by citizens and that the full range of consequences of injury control policies needs to be incorporated into evaluation research. For example, injuries might be lessened by banning the private automobile but the loss of convenient transportation services—even given expanded mass transit systems—would be considered too great by many citizens. Hence, the cost-benefit analyst seeks to translate the consequences (good and bad) of policies into a common metric (usually dollars) and pinpoint those policies that maximize net benefits (benefits minus costs).

The implications of such value conflict for the practice of evaluation research are not as disheartening as they might seem at first blush. Some proposed injury-control policies will pass or fail both the public health and cost-benefit tests. In these situations, the value conflict should be irrelevant to policy-making. As a result, it is useful for evaluation researchers to become acquainted with both frameworks and to begin to evaluate countermeasures from each perspective. For policy proposals that pass one test yet fail the other, the conflicting results can simply be reported to accountable decisionmakers and the public. For evaluators to be able to use both frameworks, they must have access to the data each framework requires. In this regard, there seemed to be a consensus among conference participants that better data should be collected on the economic costs to society of nonfatal injuries. Such information would facilitate implementation of the cost-benefit framework for evaluation.

Methodological Pluralism

The conference also addressed a more technical issue: the wide range of statistical methods currently in use to evaluate injury control interventions. While classical statistics dominates the traffic safety literature, some conference participants expressed interest in Bayesian techniques. A more fundamental debate emerged over the merits of incorporating more theoretical structure into the statistical models used to evaluate countermeasures.

Most statistical techniques currently in use to evaluate interventions retrospectively are largely atheoretical. Before-and-after or cross-jurisdictional comparisons are employed to infer what the effects of countermeasures might be. The "counterfactual" forecast—the prediction of what injury counts would have been without intervention—is based on either extrapolation of historical trends in injury counts or extrapolation from a neighboring jurisdiction. The difference between the actual postintervention injury counts and the counterfactual forecasts is ascribed to the intervention.

Some conference participants expressed a desire to see more causal factors incorporated in such statistical evaluations. Multivariate econometric methods, for example, call for introduction of intervention variables into models that also contain variables representing vehicle speed, driver age, road quality, and other covariates believed (based on theory and prior evidence) to influence injury counts. In light of the paucity of reliable data on some nonintervention variables and the absence of well-developed theories about what is important, some participants were skeptical about whether multivariate econometric approaches would give more credible results than the more atheoretical approaches. Advocates of multivariate modeling counter that evaluation research will remain on very thin scientific footing until theories of causation are devised and tested in a multivariate context.

Like the value dispute discussed earlier, the dispute about methodology is not as disheartening as it might seem at first glance. It is useful for relatively new fields of scientific inquiry to be approached from divergent methodological perspectives. The evaluation studies that employ both types of methods and arrive at similar results have a reasonable claim to being the most credible. Steps do need to be taken to foster more communication between the different methodologists so that evaluation researchers begin to develop some shared standards of quality research and acceptable data quality, even when methods differ.

Recommended Extensions of Evaluation Research

Conference participants focused their attention on three policy issues: occupant restraint use, drunk driving, and highway speeds. Obviously, these three classes of policy issues do not cover all traffic safety issues, and some classes were addressed more extensively at the conference than others. In this section, we summarize what the conference discovered about the effectiveness of interventions in these three areas and suggest some logical extensions of the evaluation literature. Our research recommendations may prove especially useful to agencies such as NHTSA and CDC which are responsible for fashioning research programs in these areas.

Occupant Restraint Policy

The recent evaluation literature on occupant restraints has focused on the consequences of mandatory seat belt wearing laws. Such laws have now been adopted in over 30 states covering almost 80 percent of the U.S. population. Evaluation researchers are interested in two basic questions:

- How effective have the laws been in each state?
- What degree of effectiveness can policymakers expect from a law with a particular set of provisions, coupled with a particular public education and enforcement program?

Most research published to date has addressed the first question, with "effectiveness" measured in lives saved. Chapter 2 by Campbell and Campbell found that belt use laws reduced highway fatalities in 24 American states by an average of 6.6 percent. In calendar years 1984 to 1986, there were an estimated 1,300 fewer fatalities in the United States than would have occurred if no states had enacted belt wearing laws. According to Campbell and Campbell, the fatality reductions are attributed to increases in belt use rates from about 10 to 35 percent in the prelaw period to anywhere from 22 to 64 percent in the postlaw period. There is a remarkable degree of variation in belt use rates, even among states with similar belt use laws.

This work can be usefully extended in two ways. First, lengthening the time period over which laws are evaluated should improve the reliability of results. Second, more research should be done to evaluate the effects of the laws on the incidence and severity of nonfatal injuries. Campbell and Campbell have made a useful start by analyzing injury data in five states (Illinois, Michigan, North Carolina, New York, and Texas) where belt use laws have been adopted.

Relatively little effort has been made so far to relate the expected effectiveness of a belt use law to its provisions and degree of enforcement. In Chapter 3, Williams and Lund report evidence that belt use rates can be increased, at least temporarily, through highly publicized police enforcement campaigns. Campbell and Campbell also present evidence that laws that permit primary police enforcement achieve higher compliance rates than laws that permit only secondary police enforcement. Yet more research needs to be done to pin down more precisely the magnitude of these relationships through use of modern statistical tools.

States vary along so many dimensions that a multivariate framework is needed to draw precise numerical conclusions about the effects of legislative provisions and enforcement on belt use rates. If precise estimates were available, they might be quite useful to state legislators who are considering bills to enact or strengthen occupant restraint legislation. The key policy levers about which information is needed are the amount of the fine, whether enforcement is primary or secondary, the per capita rate of enforcement in a state, and the extent of public information provided through various channels.

Evaluation researchers must also keep in mind that the level of enforcement (e.g., citations per capita) and the rate of belt use may be jointly determined. Although higher citation rates may induce more belt use, at some point higher usage levels will induce a decline in the citation rate. (In the extreme case where all motorists are buckled up there should be no citations, even if police engage in vigorous monitoring.) This complication requires the introduction of what economists call a simultaneous equations model, an approach that is described clearly in most applied econometrics textbooks (Kennedy, 1985).

Research and demonstration projects are also needed to identify effective methods for increasing the rate of belt use among "high-risk" groups such as teenagers and minority drivers. For example, some conference participants were optimistic that peer pressure could be tapped to increase the rate of belt use among teenagers. Minorities pose a special problem because weak belt use laws are sometimes adopted in response to fears that primary enforcement could be used by police to harass minorities. Empirical evidence on the magnitude of this problem is sorely needed.

More research also needs to be undertaken to clarify the relation between the level of belt use in a state (observed from the roadside) and the number of injuries averted. Although competent engineering studies suggest that belt use reduces fatality risk by about 45 percent (e.g., see Evans, 1986a), there are at least two theoretical reasons why this degree of safety benefit is unlikely to be achieved in the real world.

The "selective recruitment" hypothesis suggests that the people who buckle up after a law is enacted are safer drivers than those who do not comply with the law. If so, the relationship between observed belt use and percent of fatalities averted will be nonlinear. Only recently has research begun to explore quantitatively the implications of this phenomenon (e.g., Evans, 1986b).

The "risk compensation" hypothesis predicts that belt use will increase the frequency and severity of collisions by encouraging drivers to take more risks (e.g., driving faster and allowing teenagers to drive more often). Although many researchers in the traffic safety field are skeptical of this hypothesis, it is still viewed as interesting by some economists and psychologists.

The introduction of automatic restraints into the fleet in the years ahead will generate an even richer research agenda for evaluation researchers. Chapter 3 by Williams and Lund reports preliminary evidence that belt use rates vary significantly as a function of restraint design. And the simulation model presented by Graham and Henrion in Chapter 4 suggests that the relative merits of air bags and motorized automatic belts cannot be re-solved—regardless of one's value framework—without careful eval-uation of real-world experience. The volatile history of the auto-matic restraint issue suggests that policymakers are likely to revisit it again in the 1990s.

Looking into the future, it seems that evaluation researchers should be designing studies and collecting data to answer the following questions:

- Given that they are used, what are the precise injury-prevention benefits of manual belts, various automatic belt designs, and air bag systems (driver and passenger)?
- What effect do automatic restraint design features (e.g., motorized vs. nonmotorized, two-point vs. three-point, de-tachable vs. nondetachable) have on the rate of belt use?
- What effect does belt use legislation (of various sorts) have on the rate of belt use in cars with automatic restraints?
- What proportion of occupants protected by air bag systems will also wear manual safety belts?
- When economies of scale and production efficiencies are achieved, what will be the incremental cost of equipping cars with various types of automatic restraints systems (air bags and/or automatic belts)?

If evaluation researchers can provide some answers to these ques-tions, then the evidence will be available to make informed policy decisions in the 1990s.

Drunk Driving Policy

One of the conference discussants, Professor Philip Cook of Duke University, provided a useful way of conceptualizing the types of policies that are available to society to curtail drunk driving. They include the following measures (with examples):

1. Measures to reduce drinking in general
   - alcohol taxation
   - alcoholism treatment programs
   - minimum drinking age legislation
2. Measures to make drunk driving more difficult
   - limit alcohol sales on airplane flights
   - make bar servers liable
   - enact open container laws
   - redesign car ignition systems to screen inebriated drivers

3. Measures to persuade people drunk driving is a bad thing
   - public education messages
   - restrictions on advertising of alcoholic beverages
   - classes for convicted drunk drivers
   - high school education programs
4. Punitive measures to discourage people from driving while drunk
   - preconviction license suspension for those arrested for DWI
   - roadside sobriety checkpoints by police
   - 48-hour jail terms for first offenders of DWI statutes
   - "per se" laws making it a crime to drive with high BAC levels

Although the conference did not examine the effectiveness of all of these policies, Chapter 6 by Howland documents an explosion of public interest in combatting the drunk driving problem. Since the late 1970s in the United States there has been a new wave of community activism led by groups such as Mothers Against Drunk Driving. Media coverage of the issue has mushroomed, while legislative reforms at the state level have been enacted at a furious pace beginning in 1981 and 1982.

Howland points to a provocative paradox: while the policy evaluation literature in this area seems to find few unequivocal successes, there is nonetheless evidence of a substantial decline in drunk driving in the mid-1980s. The latter trend is revealed in both opinion surveys and counts of alcohol-related fatalities. Howland suggests that social norms toward drunk driving may be undergoing a fundamental change—one that is too subtle and powerful to be attributed to any particular intervention or combination of policies.

Howland's view was not shared by all conference participants. Some questioned the validity of the drunk driving indicators, especially the trends in self-reports from opinion surveys. Others questioned the permanence of the downward trend in alcohol-related fatalities, especially in light of the apparent upward trend in 1986. Still others shared Howland's view that drunk driving was on the decline but that it was attributable, at least in part, to discernible policy responses such as intensified general deterrence by police and higher minimum legal drinking ages.

The conference discussion implies that evaluation researchers need to move in at least two different directions on drunk driving policy. First, rigorous attempts need to be made to evaluate specific policies. Only those attempts that explicitly control for multiple interventions are likely to prove persuasive. Garber, in Chapter 5, highlights the difficulty of isolating the impact of one policy (minimum drinking age legislation) without formally modeling the effects of other alcohol and traffic safety policies. While drunk driving countermeasures may prove to be too collinear to make precise effectiveness estimates, the effort must nonetheless be made in a multivariate context. Second, evaluation researchers need to devote some efforts to modeling the simultaneous relationships between social norms and drunk driving policy. This will require some careful sociological theorizing and some analysis of opinion survey data. Howland, in Chapter 6, raises the interesting possibility that evaluation researchers are currently missing an important phenomenon: the effect of interventions on the social acceptability of drunk driving.

Despite the high level of public concern about drunk driving, the conference revealed that not all promising interventions have been tried. In particular, Phelps, in Chapter 7, suggests that alcohol taxation is a neglected and potentially effective policy tool for curbing drunk driving. Since the inflation-adjusted tax on alcohol has fallen by a factor of four since 1950, it is certainly appropriate to consider this policy instrument, especially in light of urgent concerns about the federal budget deficit.

From an economic point of view Phelps argues that alcohol is underpriced but by how much cannot yet be precisely determined. To resolve that uncertainty, further information is needed on:

- the relationship between drinking behavior and alcohol prices;
- the relationship between drinking behavior and driving; and
- the relationship between drinking behavior and other social costs.

Such information can probably be best gathered through detailed studies of individual behavior in which a sample of individuals is asked to keep a diary on their drinking and driving behaviors, with perhaps other information as well (to capture other social costs associated with drinking). Such a study would yield more precise information on the relative price sensitivities of different groups which would aid in setting an appropriate tax level. It would also provide information that could be used to develop more precisely targeted interventions than alcohol taxes.

Raising taxes on alcohol could in the final analysis be financially advantageous for the majority of individuals by reducing the incidence not only of traffic fatalities and injuries, but also of various medical costs. Auto and medical insurance rates might be lowered to some extent, thereby offsetting some of the increased price of alcohol. If a detailed economic analysis were to bear this out, political consensus to increase alcohol taxes might be more easily mustered.

Speed Policy

Beginning in 1987 the federal government permitted states to post speed limits as high as 65 MPH on rural interstate highways. About two-thirds of the states have done so, and Congress is now considering legislation that would permit speed limits to be relaxed on other types of highways. These changes in speed policy should provide important challenges for evaluation researchers in the years ahead.

Chapter 8 by Kamerud proposes a comprehensive research agenda for the new speed policy within the cost-benefit framework. He also presents a useful trade-off methodology that allows readers to make their own value judgments about key factors such as the monetary value of travel time and the monetary value of reduced mortality. Kamerud's approach suggests that all interstate highways should not necessarily have the same maximum speed limit.

Several items in Kamerud's research agenda deserve special recognition because they are not addressed adequately in the current evaluation literature. Some of the items concern data collection, while others involve conceptual issues.

First, greater efforts must be made to collect consistent and accurate measurements of speed on various road types. Before the recent change in policy, there were reports that some states manipulated their speed monitoring programs in order to avoid reporting excessive speeds that might trigger loss of federal highway funds. More recently, some states have considered termination of speed monitoring since the federal government no longer requires them to do so. We recommend that state and federal authorities join together in a concerted effort to collect consistent and accurate speed data. Otherwise, evaluation of changes in speed policy will be very difficult indeed.

Second, speed needs to be analyzed as a multidimensional phenomenon in evaluation research. While average speed is surely a key factor in determining the severity of injury given a crash, some attention should also be given to speed variance. It seems plausible, for example, that collision rates are positively related to speed variances on the highway, other things equal. Since changes in speed policy can—at least in principle—have opposite effects on average speed and speed variance, the two effects need to be disentangled in evaluation studies.

Third, the effects of speed policy on the trucking industry need to be analyzed with care. Conference participants noted, for example, that some large trucking companies developed a supporting infrastructure for their trucks that was synchronized to a maximum speed limit of 55 MPH. This may be one of the reasons that several large trucking companies opposed the raising of the national speed limit. Any resources devoted to adjusting infrastructures to a new policy represent a one-time cost which should be included in cost-benefit analysis of changes in the speed limit.

Fourth, the effects of alternative speed policies on vehicle wear and highway maintenance need to be measured more precisely. As important as the safety impacts of speed policy may be, evaluation researchers should also give consideration to potentially important nonsafety consequences.

Finally, policymakers have many possible policy options other than simply raising or lowering the national maximum speed limit. Simulation studies could be done to forecast the effects of having different speed limits during the day than at night, and for cars relative to trucks. Nor is there anything magic about the figures 55 and 65 MPH. Careful evaluation research might suggest 70 MPH limits on some highways and 50 MPH limits on others. At the same time, the effects of intensified police enforcement programs and improved road signs should be evaluated as a supplement or alternative to changing posted speed limits.

The Long-Term Scientific Challenge

Given the seriousness of the national injury problem, it is tempting to focus primarily on short-range research projects that will evaluate particular policy measures. The danger of this strategy is that impatience will supplant the search for fundamental knowledge. In particular, evaluation research is necessarily dependent on the advance of the basic disciplines and data systems that create knowledge about the causes of injury. Based on the conference discussion, it became apparent that there are two crucial challenges ahead in the basic scientific examination of injuries.

First, data collection is not a politically sexy topic, but there are some gaping holes in the available injury data systems that must be filled. The failure of most hospitals to record causes of injury (so-called E-codes) on hospital billing systems is a serious impediment to epidemiological investigations of the incidence and economic costs of various types of nonfatal injuries. There is also no national data system that measures the incidence of permanently disabling injuries that require long-term care and rehabilitation. Until original data collection systems are devised for nonfatal injuries, all attempts to measure the benefits of injury control policies will remain guesswork.

Second, there has been little rigorous theorizing about what behavioral processes, technological features, and environmental conditions produce observed patterns of injury. Falsifiable theories—those that generate testable predictions—need to be developed and then rigorously evaluated with available data. Theory can then be rejected, accepted, modified, and/or extended. Purely descriptive research, while valuable, is no substitute for the generation, testing, and modification of causal hypotheses. Only when evaluation researchers know how injuries are generated will they be able to make precise and accurate forecasts of the benefits of proposed interventions.

References

CRANDALL, ROBERT W., HOWARD K. GRUENSPECHT, THEODORE E. KEELER, and LESTER B. LAVE. 1986. *Regulating the Automobile.* Washington, D.C.: Brookings Institution.

EVANS, LEONARD. 1986a. "The Effectiveness of Safety Belts in Preventing Fatalities." *Accident Analysis and Prevention* 17:229–242.

———. 1986b. "Estimates of Fatality Reductions from Increased Safety Belt Use." General Motors Research Laboratories, GMR-5420.

General Accounting Office (GAO). 1976. *Effectiveness, Benefits and Costs of Federal Safety Standards for Protection of Passenger Car Occupants.* Comptroller General of the United States, Washington, D.C.

GRAHAM, JOHN D. 1984. "Technology, Behavior and Safety: An Empirical Study of Automobile Occupant-Protection Regulation." *Policy Sciences* 17:141–51.

KENNEDY, PETER. 1985. *A Guide to Econometrics.* 2d ed., Cambridge, Mass.: MIT Press.

MOYNIHAN, PATRICK. 1959. "Epidemic on the Highway." *Reporter* 30 (April).

NADER, RALPH. 1972. *Unsafe at Any Speed.* New York: Grossman Publishers.

ROBERTSON, LEON S. 1981. "Automobile Safety Regulations and Death Reductions in the United States." *American Journal of Public Health* 71:818–22.

INDEX

277